Feeling A Feeling

The Delicate Illusions of a Father and Son

By Rick Green

ISBN: 978-1-938950-76-6

Cover Art and Design: Lafe Taylor

Greater is He Publishing
9824 E. Washington St.
Chagrin Falls Ohio 44023
P O. Box 46115
Bedford Ohio, 44146

Disclaimer:

I have tried to recreate events, locales and conversations from my memories of them, and from the many interviews of Matt's friends and family, as well as his own writings. In order to maintain their anonymity, in some instances I have changed the names of individuals and places, I may have changed some identifying characteristics and details such as physical properties, occupations and places of residence.

CONTENTS

"The delicate illusions that get us through life,

can only stand so much strain."

-Hunter S. Thompson-

PROLOGUE: _____

It was a bright, sunny afternoon , on February 24, 2014. The temperature was in the upper forties, unusually mild for late winter in northeastern Ohio, and since there was no wind, it seemed even warmer. Matt Green and his longtime friend, Kevin Warner, were beginning their workout routine at the Tri-C Eastern Campus exercise facility after their Introduction to Business class was over at noon.

They'd just finished doing two sets of ten chest presses when Matt said, "I'm not feeling too good, Kev."

"Take a break," Kevin said. "I'm going to start on my pull-up sets and maybe by the time I'm finished, you'll feel a little better." He then proceeded to the pull-up bar. Matt walked away slowly, and after about ten minutes, came back looking strained.

"I'm done working out, Kev. I can't do anymore. I'm starting to feel nauseas." Kevin could see his friend wasn't his normal energetic self, so he told Matt to get dressed and go outside to get some fresh air.

"I thought that might make him feel better," he said later.

Matt went to the locker room, and while getting dressed, he noticed his breathing was getting more and more difficult. There was a tightness in his chest that he'd never felt before, and like Kevin, he thought he just needed to get outside for some air. After dressing, which seemed to him like it took forever, he went out the door of the main entrance of the campus. There were tables and benches just outside the door, and Matt went to the closest one and sat down heavily. In spite of being out in the cool air and taking several deep breaths, he still couldn't seem to get rid of the tightness he felt in his chest, and his breathing became even more labored. By this time, he knew something was definitely wrong, so he pulled out his cell phone to call his mother.

Lynda Green was sitting in her class listening to a lecture in the Women in Transition program on the Tri-C campus. She was there at the insistence of Matt, who'd persuaded her to take the class so she could get acclimated to the college environment. As she was taking notes, her cell phone began to ring noisily in her purse. Normally, she would turn off the ringer, or simply turn the phone off completely, but for some reason today, she'd neglected to do so. She was a little embarrassed because of the interruption to the class, but she somehow knew this must be urgent. She hurried out of the classroom and into the hall before answering, and when she did, she heard Matt faintly say, "Mom, I'm not feeling well. Can you come pick me up? I'm in front of the main entrance." From the sound of his voice, Lynda knew something was terribly wrong, and she immediately gathered her belongings, wasting no time, making excuses to the instructor.

All sorts of things were going through her mind as she drove the short distance from the rear to the front of the campus. What had Matt gotten into now? What did he and Kevin do that would cause Matt to get sick? She knew they liked to get high on marijuana after class, but this was different. The labored sound of Matt's voice had frightened her and made her feel uneasy. As she drove up, she saw Matt and Kevin sitting at one of the tables. As they walked to the car, she could see something wasn't right. Matt looked as if every step he took was tiring him out, and she wondered if he was going to make it to the car.

When they finally got into the car, she looked at him and said, "What's wrong Matt?"

"I had a strenuous workout, mom," was all he could say, as if that would explain everything. She pressed further.

"What do you mean 'a strenuous workout?' You don't look like that from just working out!" She then turned to Kevin, suspicion in her voice when she asked him, "What did you give Matt?" She naturally thought this was all Kevin's fault and wanted an explanation ... now!

Being put on the defensive by her question, Kevin told her they'd only smoked some weed before working out, that was all. "It wasn't anything more than that, Mrs. Green, I swear." All the while, Matt was sitting in the passenger seat, head down, not saying anything.

"How are you feeling now Matt?" she asked him. As he raised his head to answer, she saw something that made her blood run cold. His lips were blue.

"I'm not feeling too good. It must have been the workout," he said softly. Lynda drove as fast as she could, somehow knowing time was of the essence. Her baby boy was in some kind of distress, but she didn't know what to do, or how to help him. Her only thought was to get him home. Her husband Rick was there, and he would know what to do.

After what seemed like an interminable amount of time, they reached the intersection where they would drop Kevin off. As he got out of the car, Matt turned to him and said, "I'll see you, Kev." Kevin could see Matt was worse than when they'd left the school, and this worried him even more.

"Okay, Matt. I'll see you later. Go home and get some rest." He shook Matt's hand and got out of the car, and Lynda pulled off almost before he could shut the door. As he watched her go, Kevin felt an ominous dread come over him.

"I just hoped he'd be alright," he said later.

"Rick! Rick!" I was awakened from a sound sleep by the sound of Lynda's frantic voice yelling my name. "Rick, hurry up. Come, quick! Something's wrong with Matt!" The desperation in her voice made me snap out of my lethargy instantly, and I jumped up from the bed and put on my bathrobe and shoes.

"What's the matter?" I asked, expecting to see her as I came down the stairs, but she was already headed for the back door, screaming for me to hurry up.

When I came outside, I saw Matt lying face down on the ground. Lynda was hysterical and hovering over his prone body. My brother Jeryl, who apparently heard Lynda's cries for help before me, was pacing up and down the driveway with the cordless phone pasted to his ear, frantically talking to the 911 operator.

Still confused as to what was happening, I told them to turn him over so I could see his face. As they did, I could see his whole body was limp, and he was already unresponsive. He wasn't breathing, and his lips were dark blue in color. I started chest compressions, but I could tell he needed more immediate medical attention. "Where's the ambulance?" I screamed.

Jeryl said, "They're on the way!" Just as he said that, I could hear sirens getting closer in the distance. Matt was still not responding, and I was beginning to panic. Luckily, although it seemed much longer, within a few minutes of me initially getting outside, the Bedford Paramedics were rushing up the driveway with a gurney and resuscitation gear. They moved me out of the way and continued CPR as they quickly loaded him on the gurney and pushed him to the ambulance.

I was relatively sure the paramedics would help Matt and everything would turn out alright. However, Lynda wasn't of the same mind. She was crying uncontrollably and kept saying, "He's not going to make it. I just know he's not going to make it!" I tried to assure her it was going to be okay, that Matt was just having a bad reaction to whatever weed he and Kevin had been smoking. He would come out of it a little worse for the wear, but otherwise okay. Secretly, I felt like she did, but I couldn't let her see my doubts. She was inconsolable, and all I could think of was getting her to the nearby Bedford hospital as quickly as possible so she could be there with her son.

After hurriedly getting dressed, Lynda, Jeryl, and I made it to Bedford Hospital about five minutes after the ambulance. I couldn't help noticing the irony in the situation. The eerie factor was off the charts as I realized this was the same hospital where Matt was born twenty-seven years earlier. That was also a traumatic experience. He was already being attended to by the physician on duty in the emergency room, and we were told by the ER nurse to take a seat in the waiting area. "The doctor will be out to give you an update," was all she said before heading back to the emergency room.

Lynda hadn't stopped crying since we'd left the house, and it seemed as if she wasn't about to. She wouldn't sit down, but kept pacing around the waiting area, repeating, "He's not going to make it, he's not going to make it," over and over again. Nothing I said to her would make her think otherwise, and honestly, her fatalistic proclamations were starting to unnerve me. After about fifteen minutes of watching her pacing, I said, "Lynda, please sit down. The doctors are working on Matt right now. They know what they're doing. We just have to wait and keep thinking positive." Even to me, those words sounded lame, but that was all I could think to say.

She looked at me with a disdainful stare and said, "You can stay here if you want, but I can't wait here anymore. I want to go home." I felt a little upset that she didn't want to wait with me.

"What the hell?" I thought. "Why is she leaving me here to handle this alone? After all, he is *our* son." I could see she wasn't going to be dissuaded, and an argument was the last thing I wanted at a time like this. Her aunt had come to the hospital, having gotten a call from someone in the family, (how news spreads so fast in our family still boggles my mind!), and she volunteered to take Lynda home. Thankfully, my brother Jeryl said he would wait with me, so I kissed my wife and promised her I'd call as soon as I got word from the doctor.

Jeryl and I were called into the admitting station of the emergency room and were told by another nurse the doctor would be out to talk to us shortly, and then she left. We sat in silence for what seemed like forever, neither of us wanting to say anything that could possibly jinx the situation. I was thinking at the time Matt was going to be okay, and the doctor would be out soon to confirm it. Matt had been hospitalized several times in the past, usually because of his unwillingness to manage his bipolar disorder, but I knew this was not another one of his "episodes." This wasn't due to his mental illness, but whatever it was, I had to believe it wasn't life-threatening.

Finally, the doctor came out about thirty minutes later, looking solemn. I could tell the news wasn't going to be good. "How is he doctor?" I asked, rising from my chair. "Mr. Green, I'm very sorry, but your son didn't make it. He passed away without regaining consciousness. Because of his young age, I'll naturally request an autopsy be performed so you can know the cause of death. You can go in to see him now, and again, I'm truly sorry."

I sat heavily down in the chair I'd been seated in; my legs, for a moment, didn't have the strength to hold me up. I looked over at my brother, who'd collapsed on the floor after hearing the news, sobbing loudly and saying, "No, no, no!" over and over again. I helped him to his chair, still numbed by what I'd heard, my thoughts turning to Lynda, and how she would take this terrible turn of events. I feared making the call I knew I'd have to make, but it was something I couldn't avoid. I steeled myself and dialed her at home. When she answered, all I could say was, "Lynda, Matt's dead." That was all I could get out when I heard the phone drop to the floor and her anguished cries. I could hear her saying, "Oh no, my baby, my baby!" before her aunt picked up the phone and assured me she would bring Lynda to the hospital right away.

Everything after that phone call happened as if in a dream. I was led to the room where they had taken Matt's body. They left him with wires still hooked up to his chest and a tube of some sort in his mouth. He was lying on his back with his eyes closed, and for a moment, it looked like he was sleeping peacefully. As I looked closer, I could see a single tear had run down the side of his face, and that's when I lost it. I began to cry for my son.

I sat next to him, unaware that other family members were arriving at the hospital. Apparently, the word had spread like wildfire. Soon, Lynda, myself, and all of Matt's siblings were crowded around the gurney where our son, and their brother's lifeless body lay. Danielle and Angel wept silently, while John was stoic, but I could tell he was upset. Eddie cried and laid his head on Matt's shoulder. For eighteen months, Matt had lived with Eddie, and they had been inseparable. Eddie was the most affected, and he was the one who spoke first, not to us, but to Matt. "You kept talking about the "27 Club', and how famous musicians died at that age. Why did you do it Matt? Why did you have to die at 27?"

Why, indeed.

A couple of months passed before we got the results of the autopsy. The official cause of death was "thrombotic occlusion of the left anterior descending coronary artery with remote myocardial infarction, due to atherosclerotic coronary artery disease." In layman's terms, Matt died from a blood clot in one of the main arteries to the heart. The strenuous workout at the campus is what precipitated the attack. The coroner indicated Matt's arteries were hardening and narrowing because of plaque build-up. Apparently, this didn't happen overnight. The coroner said there was long-term damage due to heart disease, and because it went undetected, a heart attack could have happened at any time. Even something as simple as climbing the stairs could have triggered it.

Lynda felt a little better knowing the cause; that drugs were in no way responsible for his demise, but she was devastated. I was too, but since Matt was such a mystery to us, this only made me want to find out more about him. What was he like when he wasn't around us? What kind of man did he turn out to be?

Baltimore Sun columnist Susan Reimer wrote, "Life inside a family is a mystery, unknowable perhaps, even to its members."

Who was Matthew Thomas Green? Who was this young man that had everyone he met, including his family, asking that same question? He was a talented musician, an intellectual, a romantic, a philosopher, and bipolar. He was at once harmonious with the world, and could suddenly be contradictory.

In 2007 he wrote, "I am my own everything – mother, father, mentor, friend, foe, judge, saint, demon, whatever the circumstance calls for. I'm a psychological jack of all trades. It is quite easy to wear one thousand hats when every head they adorn is contained within the one between your shoulders."

For his family, his friends, and most importantly, for me, I wanted to take a look under some of those hats.

CHAPTER 1

Blended Family

It was a hot August day in 1986, and Lynda and I were trying to corral our brood for a group picture.

At the time, my wife, Lynda, was three months pregnant with our first child, emphasis on the word ours. We were both married once before and had kids from those relationships, but this would be our first together. We'd dated for four years before tying the knot; however, we knew from the start that if we were going to be together, our kids would have to be part of the bargain.

We had no problem with the arrangement, and we took them everywhere with us. They seemed to really enjoy each other's company, with only the occasional disagreements. After four years, we were just like a real family, so when Lynda told me she was expecting, I decided this should be made official. I put a ring on it, and we were married on July 26, 1986.

Here we were, a month later, grouped around a life-sized cutout of Sonny Crockett. For those who may not be familiar, Crockett was played by the actor Don Johnson on the hit show Miami Vice. We were big fans of the show and thought it would be cool to get a picture with the ersatz Crockett at one of the many summer events held in downtown Cleveland.

As Lynda was getting them in position for the photographer, I looked at my blended family and wondered how our new baby would fit in.

Lynda's son John was the only child she'd had with her first husband. "Johnson," as I called him, was nine years old and full of energy. He was perpetually getting into mischief, causing Lynda and I much anxiety. He had aggravated one elementary school teacher so much, she actually cried and begged us not to let him return the following year. Even at that young age, John was very opinionated and would say anything that came into his mind. Once, shortly after Lynda and I started dating, he stood in front of me with his arms folded and said, "I'll be here when you're gone." To his credit, he tried very hard to make that happen. He was fiercely loyal to his mother and acted like her little security guard, watching every move I made around her. Because she had primary custody, John was with us all the time, so I made it a point to earn his respect.

On the other hand, I had three children from my first marriage. The ex and I remained cordial after our divorce, so it was no problem for me to get them on holidays and weekends.

My oldest daughter, Danielle, was twelve years old. She was very mature for her age and considered herself "in charge" whenever Lynda and I weren't around to supervise the kids. She had no problem being the family snitch. In fact, she was quite proud of it and would say to them, "If you don't want me to tell, don't do nothing that will make me have to." She's also the most emotional, and every now and then, when something would hurt her feelings, she would need a big hug from her "daddy," while sitting in my lap. She is definitely a daddy's girl, and I'm her number one fan.

Standing next to her was my second daughter Angela, aka Angel, to her friends and family. She was ten years old and cute as a button. Her fair skin and somewhat exotic looks let me know I'd have to remain vigilant when she got into her teens and the boys took interest. Angel was the quiet one. She doesn't say much when initially meeting someone new, and it took her a while to loosen up around Lynda. Now that she was comfortable with our situation, she would talk all the time. She and Danielle had a sisterly bond that was so close, they seemed to communicate without saying a word. Where Danielle was full of personality and reveled in getting attention, Angel was more introspective. She would watch everything, and everyone, around her, silently forming her own opinions about what she saw. Later, I would listen as she'd give me her summary of whatever had transpired, and in most cases, she would be surprisingly insightful. She especially got along well with John, and she had a calming influence whenever he and Danielle got into an argument. That's not to say Angel was a pushover. On the contrary, she was as tough as they come, and had no problem "throwin' down" if the need arose.

Finally, my third child, Eddie, was six years old and already showing signs of athleticism. On any given day, you could find him doing flips around the house, climbing up on furniture, and jumping off into a perfect gymnastics roll. Eddie loved contact sports and was very physical. He and John needed constant supervision, and it was my job to keep them busy and engaged so nothing got broken, or worse, destroyed by their mischievous enthusiasm.

As we stood with Mr. Johnson, smiling and posing for the camera, I knew this family would welcome our new addition with open arms. The kids were excited, and impatient, waiting for their little brother (we'd already found out the gender a few weeks before).

The photographer snapped the picture, and since it was a Polaroid camera, we got it back right away. I looked at the somewhat grainy black and white photo and saw six smiling faces, (seven if you count Crockett), and wondered just how our new charge would fit into this mixture of diverse personalities.

None of us knew what our future as a family would be with the new baby, but eager with anticipation, and fingers-crossed hope, we were ready… or so we thought.

CHAPTER 2

January 6, 1987

"Come on, Green, show us whatcha got!" came the beer-soaked words of my friend from my job's bowling league. I had two strikes in the tenth frame of our finals match. One more would clinch a win, and also a sizeable jackpot for me. I was totally focused on the business at hand. I would not be denied; a strike was imminent.

I was just about to make my approach to the line for my final shot when I heard a voice frantically calling my name. "Rick, Rick!" I was startled out of my concentration by my teammate, Liz Billingsley. I was pissed off and ready to give Liz a good dressing down until I saw the frightened look on her face.

"What's wrong, Liz?" I asked, starting to get a little worried myself.

Liz, who had walked with my wife Lynda to the snack bar not more than five minutes ago, said, "Something's happened to Lynda. She's passed out over there, and they're calling an ambulance right now! I'm not kidding, Rick. Hurry!",she insisted, and ran back to the snack bar.

Lynda was eight months pregnant, and her pregnancy to this point had been fairly uneventful, the usual pains and discomforts notwithstanding. However, her due date wasn't for another month, so her passing out so suddenly caused me to go into a panic.I muscled my way through the crush of onlookers yelling, "Let me through. That's my wife!" The crowd separated like I imagine it looked when Moses parted the Red Sea, and I found Lynda on the floor of the snack bar, with her eyes partially opened, her breathing labored.

Even though her eyes were half closed, I could see the parts that should have been white were solid red. It looked as if all the vessels had ruptured, making the dark irises look like they were floating in blood. I was shocked into immobility by the sight of her, so thank goodness someone had the presence of mind to call 911 as soon as it happened.

In just a few minutes from the time I'd reached Lynda, the Bedford first responders were rolling a gurney into the snack bar. I was moved away by a pair of strong, but gentle hands from Lynda's side, and I vaguely heard someone say, "We're paramedics. Please give us room." I began to understand the gravity of the situation and slowly came to the realization that something could happen to my wife, or our unborn child, or both.

As they were simultaneously working on her vital signs and loading her onto a gurney, I thought back on anything I could remember. Anything at all that may have given me a sign something was wrong. Nothing came to mind. Our day started out typical, with both of us going to work, agreeing to meet at the bowling alley afterwards. Nothing out of the ordinary.As I rode in the ambulance watching one paramedic attach an IV to her arm, and the other one looking into her eyes with a small flashlight, my mind was racing. What's wrong? What about the baby? What about Lynda? Will they be alright? How far are we from the hospital? My anxiety level was starting to rise when the ambulance came to an abrupt stop, and the back doors were flung open. A contingent of medical staff descended on Lynda as they hurriedly removed the gurney from the conveyance.

She was whisked away to the emergency room for evaluation, while someone from the hospital's admissions office pulled me away to sign those ubiquitous insurance forms. Afterwards, a nurse came to me and said, "The doctor attending to your wife needs to speak with you. He'll be out to see you in a minute."

In about forty-five seconds, a tall, rugged-faced man in green scrubs, came in and introduced himself as the emergency room doctor. Then he said, "Mr. Green, your wife has something called eclampsia. In a nutshell that means her blood pressure has spiked to a dangerously high level. Both she and the baby are at risk."

"Eclampsia?" I said, "What the hell is that?" The doctor was very professional and seemed not to notice my agitation. His voice was calm, but filled with urgency when he said, "Mr. Green, I have to be totally upfront with you. Because her blood pressure is so high and can't be quickly stabilized, both she and your unborn child are in danger." His words didn't quite register with me, and just as I was about to ask more questions, he continued. "If we work to help your wife, the blood supply could be sufficiently compromised to cause brain damage to the fetus, or worse. However, we could perform an emergency C-section, which will almost guarantee the child's safety, but without first stabilizing your wife's blood pressure, she could have a stroke and expire during the surgery. I don't envy the position you're in Mr. Green, but you don't have a lot of time. I have to go back to check on your wife, but a nurse will be out in the next few minutes to get your decision. I'm sorry," he said, and then he was gone.

My mind was racing with indecision. Should I save Lynda, the love of my life, my constant companion, my soulmate? Or should I let them save the baby, whose only chance at life was swiftly ticking away as the minutes flew by. What should I do? Please God, help me decide, I prayed.

Lynda and I had children from a previous marriage, and we worked hard to raise them in an environment as loving and nurturing as possible. Even though I didn't have primary custody of my three, they often spent weekends and holidays with Lynda, her son John, and me. They got along well together, and we always tried to foster love and respect for others among our kids. I also knew how excited they were when they found out Lynda was pregnant, so I knew they would love him just as much as they loved and cared for each other.

Just then, the nurse came back and said, "Mr. Green, the doctor wants your decision right away. Your wife's blood pressure is getting higher and we don't have much time." At that moment, I knew what I should do.

"Save the baby," I said. "I think that's what Lynda would want too."

The nurse hurriedly left to inform the doctor, while another nurse told me to put on scrubs, which I did in record time. I was then ushered into the operating room. What I was witnessing could only be called controlled chaos. The doctor was giving orders to the nurses as the anesthesiologist administered the drugs that put Lynda mercifully to sleep. IV's were in both her arms and her entire body was covered in a white sheet that only exposed her swollen belly.

I watched, fascinated but horrified, as the doctor expertly made an incision across the lower part of Lynda's stomach.

Blood and all kinds of unknown tissue sprang forth from the gaping wound, but he wasn't done yet. I heard him say to one of the nurses, "Suction!" One of the nurses pulled what looked like a tiny vacuum cleaner hose from out of nowhere, and started sucking the blood away for the doctor to get a clear view. Then he said, "Fresh scalpel!" Another nurse slapped one into his hand, and he started to cut Lynda some more.

"What, more cutting?" I thought. I had just watched him slit open my wife's stomach, making an opening that seemed to me big enough to deliver twins, and now he was going to cut her some more? Everyone was talking; the doctor barking orders as he proceeded to cut, the nurse monitoring Lynda's blood pressure and vital signs, all the while relaying what she saw to the doctor. All this I barely heard, watching transfixed, as the doctor slowly removed the baby from his mother's womb.

The baby wasn't crying initially, making me think, "Oh God, he's not making any noise. I've lost him, too." However, as the nurse carried him to the opposite side of the operating room to clean him up, I could hear him start to cry, and my heart rejoiced! "My son is alive," I said, "Thank God he's alive!" My happiness was short lived as I returned my attention to my wife, whom I was certain was about to die.

I kissed my son and was going over to do the same to Lynda when the nurse manning the blood pressure monitor said, "Doctor, her blood pressure is starting to lower!"

The doctor said, "Keep monitoring her BP and let me know if it starts going higher again." He was stitching her stomach as he was talking, never losing his concentration as he worked feverishly to close her up."Still going down," the nurse said. By this time, the doctor had completed his repair work on Lynda's stomach and had joined the nurse watching the BP monitor. I didn't know whether to go to Lynda and try to hold her hand as she took what I was sure would be her last breath, or to go over to our new baby and hold him in my arms to assuage my fears of losing my wife, and his mother.

Suddenly, I heard the doctor say, "Amazing!"

I turned to him and asked, "What's going on, doctor?" afraid to hear his answer.

"Well, Mr. Green, it would seem your wife's blood pressure is stabilizing on its own. I've never seen anything quite like it. I've never seen a spiked BP reading lower so fast after a full blown eclampsia episode. However, she's still not out of the woods. We'll take her to the ICU for further monitoring to make sure she doesn't have a recurrence of the spiking, but as of now, the immediate danger has passed."

I wasn't quite ready to believe what I was hearing, which is when I asked, "Is she going to live?"

The doctor looked at me with compassionate eyes and said, "I believe so, but we won't know if there will be any long term damage from her blood pressure being so high. It could have an effect on some of her brain functions. We'll know more in the next 24 to 48 hours." Then he said, "Your wife and baby are very lucky, Mr. Green. It looks like you'll both be able to enjoy life with your new son."

My son... I'd almost forgotten about him. In the tense moments immediately after his birth, I had been so focused on Lynda that he temporarily slipped my mind! He was no longer crying, and was comfortably wrapped in hospital blankets. The nurse gave him to me, and as I watched them wheeling his mother's gurney to the ICU, I heard a small whimper.

Looking at him, so small and fragile in my arms, I was overwhelmed with emotion and a profound relief. I had made the right decision. I was pretty sure Lynda was going to be alright, and now that I was holding this five-pound, eight-ounce bundle of joy, I somehow knew he would be okay too. I said a silent prayer of thanks, and then formally introduced myself to my son.

"Hello, Matthew Thomas Green," I said. "I'm your dad. Welcome to the family." I sat down with him cradled in my arms and wept tears of relief. It was January 6, 1987, and with this birth, Lynda and I had to change our initial thoughts on how to raise a child. This kid was about to take us on a wild ride... I just wish I had fastened my seatbelt.

CHAPTER 3

Matt and Me

From the time he was brought home from Bedford Hospital, Matt's life and mine seemed destined to be, for better or worse, inextricably intertwined.

I don't think we were consciously aware, and we definitely never admitted as much; it just seemed the "powers-that-be" deemed us to be tethered for life.

Right after Matt was born, Lynda was kept in the hospital for a few weeks following his traumatic delivery. She was still being monitored for residual damage from her eclampsia episode, but she also began to suffer postpartum depression. I had to be the one to keep up with his needs for the first six weeks of his life. Even after she was well enough to come home, she still wasn't able to keep up with the daily routine I'd established for his feeding and changing.

After a month of trying to look after Lynda and making sure Matt was attended to, I was exhausted. I had to admit to myself that I couldn't "do it all." I finally broke down and sent out the S.O.S to the one person I knew would answer unconditionally. My hero came in the form of my mother, Willie Lee Green, the big-hearted matriarch of our family from Fort Worth, Texas. "Mama" had been divorced from my dad for fifteen years when Matt entered the picture. She'd moved back to her home town since then, but always longed to come back to Cleveland to be with her grandchildren. She was also dreading the brutal heat imminent during the Texas summers, and the thought of the milder temperatures in the 'Land' was quite appealing. "Give me 'til the end of the week!" she said gleefully. "I'll see you on Saturday!"

She quickly came into our small apartment and went to work organizing the mess I'd accumulated for the baby, and putting him on a much better schedule than the one I'd come up with. She not only kept pace with Matt's erratic schedule, but she was able to make life a lot easier for Lynda, who deeply appreciated her mother-in-law's help.

When Matt was six months old, my son Eddie, who was six years old at the time, said, "Dad, what's wrong with his eyes?" I looked over at him sitting on the couch holding Matt, and staring intensely into his face.

"What do you mean, 'what's wrong with his eyes?'" I asked as I picked up Matt and held him so I could get a closer look at his eyes.

In a small, somewhat frightened voice, Eddie said, "They won't stop moving." Matt had just woken up from a nap, so I figured he was just trying to get his young eyes accustomed to the light in the room. However, as I watched more closely, I began to notice side-to-side movement in both eyes, as if they were swinging on an invisible pendulum, even when he was looking straight at me.

I looked in Matt's eyes for ten minutes straight, and not once in that time did the movement stop. I started to become alarmed. I had no idea what could be causing this to happen; I immediately thought of residual damage due to his traumatic birth months earlier. Then, I started looking to lay blame on someone. Why hadn't mama noticed this before? We'd just taken him for a follow-up visit to the pediatrician, and all he said was, "The baby's coming along just fine." Why didn't he notice it?

I was becoming angrier by the minute when Eddie, whom I'd totally forgotten about, tapped me on the shoulder and said, "Dad, is Matt going to be blind?" The question jolted me from my festering thoughts, and I could see Eddie was genuinely upset about his brother. My heart broke for him, and I quickly lost my anger.

I told him to sit down with me on the couch, putting my arm around him while still holding Matt, and said, "No son, Matt's not going to be blind. Look, he reaches for my finger when I hold it in front of his face." As if on cue, Matt grasped my finger, and in one swift movement, put it in his mouth. I could see Eddie relax somewhat, but he still didn't look convinced, until I told him to give it a try. He tentatively put his finger about a foot from Matt's face. He released my soggy finger from his mouth and reached with his other hand for his brother's proffered digit. Eddie giggled with delight as Matt happily bit down on his finger with a toothless clamp.

I left Eddie and Matt in the living room to play, the eye movements temporarily forgotten, but I knew I'd have to tell Lynda about our discovery, and it would have to be done gently. She was doing much better; she'd actually gone back to work at the bank a few weeks prior, but I wasn't too sure how she would handle this new revelation. I decided to wait until Matt's next doctor visit, which was a week away, to broach the subject. I wasn't even going to tell my mother, since she apparently hadn't noticed anything up to now, and in her defense, neither did anyone else in the family.

If it hadn't been for Eddie's perceptiveness, we may have never known about Matt's eyes—at least not as soon as we did. I watched Lynda and my mom interact with Matt the following week, and they didn't seem to notice his eye movements. They played with him and did all the things one does with a new baby, but they carried on as if there was nothing wrong. Even John, who was ten at the time and with Matt on a daily basis, never said anything about his brother's eyes. My anxiety level grew when it was time for me to get the girls for a weekend sleepover. I knew how observant Danielle and Angel could be, Danielle especially, but they had been around him for six months and, up to now, hadn't said a word. Eddie, bless his heart, seemed to understand my need for secrecy and didn't say anything to his siblings about what he'd noticed. Matt's next doctor visit couldn't come fast enough!

The day finally came for us to take Matt to his appointment. As we drove to the office, I looked over at Lynda sitting quietly in the passenger seat, and then glanced back at Matt sleeping soundly in his car seat behind her. I relished the peaceful ride but was a little anxious, anticipating the ride home. I had no way of knowing how Lynda would react, but I said a silent prayer the news wouldn't cause her to have a relapse into depression.

Once there, I waited until the doctor did his examination and declared all was well in Matt's development. "Everything looks good," he said. "He's still a little underweight, but that should rectify itself once he gets on solid food."

Lynda looked happy with the news, but I felt a twinge of fear as I said, "Dr., I've noticed a constant movement in the baby's eyes. Did you see that during his examination?"

I caught a quick glimpse of Lynda as I spoke, looking intently into Matt's face while she held him. The doctor frowned and said, "Let me take a look." He took Matt from

Lynda and sat him on his lap. He raised a finger in front of his eyes, but just out of reach. We all looked closely as Matt reached up for his finger. In the past week I'd done this so much, Matt automatically grabbed any finger and would chew on it. His little mind must have thought it was a game of some sort. However, as he reached for the doctor's finger and found he couldn't get it, he began to fret and cry, never taking his eyes off the finger. And his eyes never stopped moving. In fact, when he got upset, they moved even more!

The doctor handed him back to Lynda and said matter-of-factly, "It seems he has some sort of nystagmus, although I can't say for sure. I do think it's something that should be looked into further, so I'm going to give you a referral to a pediatric ophthalmologist so you can get a more definitive diagnosis."

I was waiting for Lynda's reaction upon hearing this, but she seemed to be as calm as ever, and said, "Thank you doctor. We'll make an appointment for him as soon as possible." Even though she was outwardly calm, I could see in her eyes she was struggling to maintain her composure. I loved her more than ever at that moment. I admired her strength, and her refusal to let this new development overwhelm her. I made a vow to myself right then. *I* would be the one to handle whatever complications arose where Matt was concerned. I was not going to let her fragile emotions be assaulted by worry for her baby.

***

Fast forward to 1993. Matt is six years old and wearing glasses. We'd taken him to be examined by numerous specialists in pediatric ophthalmology, and every one of them said Matt had pendular nystagmus. They explained it was a congenital condition, which caused the eye movements. There was no cure for it, but because he was so young, we wouldn't know if corrective lenses would help or not until he was old enough for school.

By now, the family had grown accustomed to Matt's eyes. We all knew about his condition, and it didn't seem to affect how his siblings reacted to him. However, I was still constantly watching him, trying to gauge how well he could see. If there was any tell-tale sign, I'd notice as he grew into school age. I was afraid he'd be ridiculed (children can be cruel in kindergarten) because of his eye movements. So Lynda and I made sure we checked often to see if we saw him having difficulty because of it. We wanted to give him every advantage he needed to overcome his nystagmus.

By 1993, Matt had not only gone to, and passed from, kindergarten, he enjoyed every day he was there. Also, my earlier fears about him being ridiculed were unfounded because, according to his teacher, Matt was very popular with his classmates *because* of his eyes! "No one makes fun of him, Mr. Green," she said, laughing. "In fact, they think his eyes are kind of cool."

The glasses Matt was wearing were prescribed by his optometrist, with the caveat we'd probably have to buy him new glasses every year until he was well into elementary school. "This may help him for now, but because his eyes are still developing, you should have him re-examined every year. The prescription will probably have to be changed by then."

We didn't know for sure if the glasses worked or not because Matt said they helped about as often as he'd say they didn't. He'd watch television and take them off sometimes. Other times, he'd have them on. We just left him alone and kept a close watch on him. Since he always held books closer to his face when he was reading, (that was with, or without glasses), seeing him do that wasn't of much concern.

Since he loved school, and since he didn't seem to have a confidence problem, I decided not to be so much of a "hover parent" where Matt was concerned. I had watched over him, and been his staunch supporter, since his birth. I never forgot his traumatic introduction to the world, and I never forgot my vow to not let Lynda be worried about our son. I had no regrets about that, but I was finding it hard to let Matt grow up. I still remembered him as that cute little premature baby who needed me for everything — not this still cute, but more noticeably independent, first-grader. He'd taken to saying, "I can do it myself, daddy!" when I tried to help him tie his shoe. Or "You don't have to watch me get dressed anymore. I don't need any help." I guess he was getting a little annoyed by my constant monitoring.

"Sorry Matt. I forget you're a big boy now," I'd say and shut his bedroom door.

All things considered, Matt had done relatively well with his eye problem. He made adjustments at home, and we made arrangements with his teachers to have him seated in the front of the classroom so he could see things a little better. Other than that, Matt was developing into a healthy, bright, confident child, and the family adored him. Everything was going great.

Little did I know at the time, these early years with Matt would be the calm before the storm.

CHAPTER 4

Matt, Sam, and the Guitar

As a young child, from the age of five to about nine years old, Matt was a happy, well-adjusted kid. He enjoyed going to school and learning new and different things, and showed an early interest in reading and writing. He started his first journal when he was six.

He was always inquisitive and would often ask me how things worked, like clocks, radios, and TVs. At his school, he was put into accelerated classes because, as it was explained to me by his first grade teacher, he needed more "engaging" instruction.

When he was eight years old, one of his elementary school counselors asked me to come for a conference to talk about Matt's progress. I came at the appointed time, and the counselor took me to his office and asked me to be seated. He opened a manila folder that was lying on his desk and said it was Matt's file.

I was a little worried. I didn't think Matt had been a bad student, and he always had good things to say when we would ask him about his day at school. "How's he doing?" I asked.

He looked up from the papers he'd been scanning and said, "According to his progress reports, he's doing quite well. His teacher says he's one of her best students. But that's not the reason for this conference."

I tensed up, waiting for the news that I somehow knew would be bad. The counselor continued, "Mr. Green, recently our students were given a series of aptitude tests to give us an indication of their learning potential and abilities. Matthew's scores are the equivalent of a person with an I.Q. of 139."

All I could do was nod my head, but I said nothing. I didn't know what this new information implied, but I was sure it had to be significant. I knew Matt was smart for his age, but I had no clue as to his real intellect, nor how it would play out in the years to come. Besides, I was certain whatever tests they used to come up with that score had to be flawed in some way. "How can an eight-year-old be accurately tested for I.Q. in the first place?" I thought to myself.

However, I had to admit, the prospect of raising a child with above-average intelligence intrigued me. I was imagining Matt becoming a doctor or lawyer, the first in the family.

With his early interest in electronics, I thought of him being an engineer of some sort, or even a research scientist. The possibilities for a highly intelligent child were astronomical, but because Matt was *my* son, the prospects were limitless!

I had to ask the counselor what this meant for Matt's continued education at their school. He indicated Matt's teachers had already been aware of his potential and had adjusted his curriculum to accommodate his advanced learning capabilities. He also told me be prepared to be constantly vigilant in his upbringing. Then, he said cryptically, "His natural curiosity will cause him to want answers to questions you and your wife may not be able, or willing, to give."

Before I could ask him to explain further, he said, "You see, Mr. Green, in my experience with highly intelligent children, I've found the parents are the ones who have the most anxiety. These children have a propensity to sometimes make unwise choices in an effort to satisfy their curiosity about all things, as they get older. I don't want you to be overly concerned at this point. I would suggest you find things outside of school he likes, and allow him to explore whatever interests him, within reason, of course. As long as you keep him mentally stimulated, there should be very few problems."

With that, he ended our meeting. I thanked him for updating me, and for his advice, and left the school. As I walked to my car in the school parking lot, I decided to keep a close eye on Matt's development over the next few years. If Lynda and I had to raise a very intelligent child, we were going to have to step up our game to keep his mind occupied. So our job would be to make sure he realized, while he was being "mentally stimulated," no matter how smart he was, we were still his parents. He would have to respect our rules.

From that day forward, I watched how Matt progressed in school, and at home. All through his elementary school years, Matt made excellent grades. He was a regular on the Honor and Merit rolls and was even named "Student of the Week" twice by the school faculty. He needed very little help with his assignments, seemingly able to retain information after hearing, or reading, the instructions once or twice. He loved to read and even asked for a library card at the age of nine, which he kept current, and used often, into adulthood.

Good grades and being an avid reader didn't necessarily mean our son had an above average I.Q. I was beginning to think I was right about the "test" being inaccurate. There was nothing exceptional, from my perspective, that persuaded me we had a potential "genius" on our hands. I'd just have to keep watching him and maybe something would show up.

Then came the summer of 1998. School was out, and since we both worked full time, we had to get Matt involved in some sort of summer program that would keep him engaged but active. There was the Southeast YMCA just a few miles from our apartment, and Lynda knew there was a summer activities program for the neighborhood kids to attend while their parents were at work. She decided that would be the best place for Matt since they not only had games and field trips, but also things to do that would be physically challenging. Our plan was to have Matt exhausted and ready to wind down by the time we picked him up.

While attending the Y's summer camp session, he met a youngster who would eventually become his best and closest friend, Sam Sizemore. Sam was twelve years old at the time, and Matt was a year younger. Their friendship would last for the next sixteen years. Sam and Matt hit it off right from the beginning, and before that long hot summer was over, they had become almost inseparable.

Sam was an unassuming kid of average build, with a shock of unruly dark brown hair, and penetrating eyes. Even then, Sam had a rebellious streak that wouldn't allow convention to dictate his self-expression. He would change his appearance at the drop of a hat and was perfectly comfortable with the stares he would get from his unusual transfigurations.

His hair was typically what would be noticed first. From blue to green, from long to short, and even spiked into a Mohawk, Sam's look was uniquely his own, and Matt found this especially fascinating. As a youngster, Sam would dress unconventionally in whatever style he felt fit his mood at the time. When he and Matt were feeling "rad," they would don their leather jackets with spikes or studs attached, and would walk around downtown Bedford, the ultimate odd couple, enjoying the looks coming from shop owners and passersby.

According to Sam, their connection, initially, was their love of music. Even though Matt was younger, his knowledge of artists such as the Rolling Stones and the Beatles, to name a few, intrigued Sam. Plus, Matt was like no other black kid Sam knew at the time. "He seemed to be more comfortable around white kids," Sam remembered. "I don't think the music he liked appealed to black kids, and Matt wasn't into Hip-Hop."

They would alternate weekend sleep-overs between our house and Sam's, and it was after one of these that Matt came home asking us to buy him a guitar. It turned out Sam was learning to play, and Matt thought it would be cool to learn too, so he and Sam could play together. At eleven years old, I just thought it was a phase he was going through. He'd try it for a while and then go on to whatever else would tickle his fancy. However, I was secretly hoping it would be more than a passing interest. You see, I played a little piano and was a lead singer in a couple of groups when I was younger, and I always wanted my musical genes to somehow show themselves in at least one of my kids. Unfortunately, none of them had shown an interest, or inclination, to learn how to play an instrument.

Plus, I knew buying a guitar would be a monetary investment I didn't want wasted, so before I purchased one, I needed to know just how committed Matt would be. "Listen, Matt, if I buy you a guitar, will you promise to do what's necessary to be at least half-way good at it?" I asked. I was setting the bar pretty low since I didn't want to put too much pressure on him.

He looked me straight in the eye and said, "I promise, dad. In fact, I promise to practice every day until I get more than 'half-way good'. I'll be all the way good." I still wasn't fully convinced. What sounded like total conviction to him sounded like a child's bravado to me. I was still worried about squandering good money on whimsy. However, I knew he and Sam were pretty close, and if Sam had a guitar and was practicing, Matt would most definitely want to do the same. So I broke down and bought a starter guitar and amplifier at the local Guitar Center for $100. I figured if he didn't do as he said, I'd only be out a C-note. Hell, I might even pick it up and give it a try myself if he lost interest.

I was pleasantly surprised when he actually did keep his promise. He practiced daily, amp cranked up to ear-splitting proportions, playing scales and strumming chords that initially sounded awful, but within a few weeks, sounded a little better. He'd also take his equipment to the aforementioned sleepovers. I later learned from Sam's mother, Shannon, they sounded as cacophonous as Matt at home... only times two!

It was during this time I began to notice a shift in Matt's focus. This was the first time I'd seen him this obsessed with something. He used to enjoy skateboarding every day. He spent hours on end, scaring the shit out of his mother and I while trying to do various tricks and maneuvers. He'd even been instrumental in having a skate park built by leveraging his friendship with a kid whose father was a Bedford city councilman. Now, the skateboard was collecting dust as he practiced his guitar diligently every day. When he wasn't playing, he was reading everything he could get his hands on about the guitar and how to improve his technique.

His grades never suffered while he was learning to play. School work, for him, was a bothersome, but necessary distraction. It had to be done before he could get back to his guitar. Our agreement was school first, guitar second. That was non-negotiable. He'd dutifully complete all his homework, let us check it, and head to his room to practice.

He started listening to old Beatles and Rolling Stones records, over and over, while trying to emulate what he heard on his guitar. The scratchy music coming from the speakers of an old throwback record player, combined with the amplified twangs of Matt's Stratocaster, was reason for some serious Tylenol usage in the Green household!

There were times we'd have to make him stop practicing so he could eat dinner. He'd wolf it down in five minutes, or less, and go right back to his room to practice some more. This used to worry his mother. Matt had always had a healthy appetite and would never miss her delicious home-cooked meals. Now, it was as if his appetite had been lulled into stasis by the melodies coming from his guitar. I couldn't believe how focused he was on mastering his instrument, and I couldn't be happier or more proud.

Within a few months, the sounds coming from my son's room went from screeching noise to actual semblances of real rock and roll music. He was able to play along with the Beatles and Rolling Stones records almost as well as John Lennon or Keith Richards. Wow! My boy's gonna be a musician! I was elated to know I finally had a child that not only wanted to play music, but was obsessed with it.

In the span of a year, Matt had mastered all those Beatles and Rolling Stones records. Now, he'd moved on to Mott the Hoople, Bob Dylan, and just about any music he'd hear on the local rock and roll stations. His record collection began to grow, and with it, his guitar playing repertoire. His ability to listen to a tune once or twice and play it back almost exactly was pretty impressive. He would become completely absorbed in whatever genre of music he was trying to play, to the point of researching the lives of the artists who made the music.

I could see now the "above average intelligence" the counselor had told me about years before was indeed showing itself. Matt may not become a doctor or lawyer, but I was completely satisfied with the knowledge he could be a guitar virtuoso someday. I imagined him playing to packed venues all over the world, and me, backstage, beaming proudly at my son. I was a happy man! What he needed now was formal training. I decided it was time for him to take lessons from a professional instructor.

Like a man seeing his son get drafted to play a professional sport, I was just as proud. Matt was going to take us to the promised land!

CHAPTER 5

Slimmy Hendrix

By the spring of 1999, Matt had convinced us to move to Bedford, Ohio, a quiet suburb of Cleveland that just happened to be where his best friend Sam resided. Since the beginning of their budding friendship, Sam had been taking him around the neighborhood and introducing him to people, some of whom would eventually become Matt's life-long friends. In the process, Matt was becoming more and more inclined to be around kids with interests more in tune with his own. In most cases, they would be the white kids.

Matt used to say the black kids he knew would sometimes ridicule him for not liking hip hop music, and because he wore clothes that were different from theirs. He said he didn't feel comfortable around them most of the time, notwithstanding his family. "They just don't get me dad," he would often say. "With Sam and his friends, I don't have to be afraid to talk about the kind of music I like because they like it too. Even my own brothers and sisters make fun of my music!" he'd say incredulously.

We had been looking to buy our first house in an area that would be conducive to raising a precocious and opinionated twelve-year-old. Also, we wanted Matt to be in a decent school system, one that wasn't about to be put on "Academic Watch," a term used to describe a school district that was on the verge of a state takeover, like the one we were moving from. We had already narrowed our search down to three communities, Bedford being one of them, but Matt's friendship with Sam sealed the deal.

On Memorial Day weekend 1999, we moved into our house at 109 Southwick Drive. It was, a beautiful old brick Tudor-style home, built in 1927. Lynda and I loved the fireplace in the living room, and the fact it had a finished basement, with three bedrooms on the second floor. The street itself was lined with well-kept lawns, and the flower beds of most of them were brilliant with brightly colored flowers.

Matt quickly claimed the bedroom at the back of the house, with windows looking out over the backyard. He happily carried his boxes filled with books to his room, and started arranging them on the built-in bookshelves that were put in by the previous owners. We had no doubt we'd made the right choice in moving here, and we felt comfortable right from the start.

By summer of that year, we had settled into our new home, and since Matt was out of school, (he would start junior high in the fall), we felt it was time for him to take guitar lessons with a professional instructor. He'd taught himself to play just about everything he heard on his records, but I knew if he was to become even more proficient, he would need to have formal training.

Inwardly, I was living vicariously through my son because I'd always dreamed of becoming an entertainer. I'd been a member of several bands and singing groups over the years, but it never amounted to much more than a few bucks and free beers at the spots we played in. I just knew, with my help, and his talent, we could make both our dreams come true!

He was excited when I told him I'd found an excellent music school in Cleveland Heights that had a guitar instructor who was already playing in a band. His name was Matthew Abroms, and because they had the same first name, Matt felt it was a perfect match. I took him to his lessons religiously twice a week, and he seemed to enjoy coming home showing us what he'd learned. He was taught to read music and use proper fingering on the frets of his guitar to make chord progressions faster and more seamlessly. He was given sheet music to practice at home, and by his next lesson, he'd have it down pat. I was truly amazed at how far he had come with his playing. It was like he was a sponge and soaked up everything he was being taught. Even Lynda would comment on how good his music sounded when he practiced in his room. Matt had been taking lessons twice a week for six months when the instructor Abroms pulled me to the side and said, "Mr. Green, I can't teach your son anymore." I was surprised to hear this, but I said nothing. I just looked at him and waited for him to continue. When he saw I wasn't responding, he continued, "Matt has mastered the fundamentals of playing the guitar at an amazing speed. Some of the more intricate chord progressions he's picked up faster than any of my other students, and some of them have been taking lessons much longer than he has. He's playing whole songs he hears for the first time in just a few takes. He tells me the assignments I give him to practice at home are too easy, and he wants me to give him more challenging material."

Finally, I said, "Well, why don't you give it to him?" He gave a wan smile and said, "Because the stuff he's asking for is beyond my realm of expertise. He needs more advanced training."

He said he could recommend someone, but I said I'd have to discuss it with Matt first. I wanted to hear his side of the story. When we got into the car heading home, I asked him how the lesson went. He was quiet for a moment as he looked distractedly out the window. Then he turned to me and said, "It was okay, but it's getting to be boring. I keep asking him to give me harder music to practice, and he keeps saying what

I'm being taught is all he has." That's when I decided to tell him what Abroms said. After I'd relayed our conversation he just said, "That's okay dad, I don't need any more lessons. I'll just keep teaching myself." The finality in his voice let me know it would be useless to bring up another instructor, so I just let it pass. We continued the rest of the ride home in silence.

From that day forward, he would play his guitar for hours at a time, night and day, until he became proficient enough to write and play his own music, and true to his word, he never took another lesson.

Matt had always wanted to be in a band; he and Sam had been practicing together for most of the year, so those two forming a band was an obvious progression. I encouraged him whole-heartedly, buying him new guitars when he'd worn out his previous ones, some so beat up they couldn't be salvaged by re-stringing. I fantasized about his finding a good cover band, playing the music he was exposed to at home: Motown, R&B, maybe a little jazz. Man, I would LOVE going to one of those gigs!

But alas, that was not to be.

As expected, he formed a band with Sam called the Flying Squirrels in 2000. They practiced frequently, and even wrote a few songs. However, the first "official" band Matt joined, at the tender age of 15, was a punk rock group called the Subverts in 2002. The band consisted of Matt on lead guitar, Tony Furino on drums, and Mitch Culver on bass. The Subverts introduced me to a counter-culture I'd only imagined really existed, but it was the beginning of Matt's transformation into the person he would ultimately become.

CHAPTER 6

Punk'd

"The Punk years of my life were some of the most memorable and timeless. The places, faces, and events, shaped me into who I am more than anything else that I have been through in my life. To me, punk was the holy grail of teenage counter-cultures, and now that I think about it, my transformation from average pre-pubescent adolescent into a full-fledged, drinking, smoking, pseudo-anarchist gutter punk, was actually a very natural, and logical, progression or process."

- Matt Green -

Matt had been an avid skateboarder for a couple of years by the time we'd moved to Bedford. He'd gotten pretty good at it too, although his mother and I worried about him getting injured; he'd hurt his arm once while trying a kick-jump. We didn't discourage him in any way from doing it. We wanted him to meet new friends, and we knew skateboarding to him was like Lynda and I having backyard-socials with our neighbors, which we did. Matt already had friends in Bedford before moving there. The kids he hung around were skaters too, and they'd come by to get Matt, dressed in the outfits that identified them as skaters — printed t-shirts, straight-legged jeans, and Vans shoes, "Specially designed for skateboarding," he would say.

Matt's initial meeting with Tony Furino was at a mutual friend's house around 2000. This friend played Dungeons and Dragons with Matt, and Tony would go by, at their invitation. They always talked about how cool it was. Tony would tell me later, "I went over there just to see how lame it was, and it turns out, I hated it!" His reaction must have been noticeable because sometime later, Matt informed him of his demeanor. "He told me I made a horrible first impression," Tony said.

Their next encounter was at the neighborhood skate park, which they both frequented, some years later. Tony was four years older than Matt, but because the skaters in Bedford were few, their meeting could be considered inevitable. Everyone in that scene knew, or was acquainted with, each other. Skaters in Bedford were also acquainted with the Bedford punks, and would often commiserate about the social injustices of society. The skaters and punks were also the ones who seemed to be the "outsiders." As Tony would tell me later, "We were sort of the misfits. We weren't like the jocks or the preppy kids in school, so we kind of gravitated to each other."

After Matt had been playing guitar for a few years, he got back in touch with Tony, who by now had already formed his band, the Subverts. He and his friend, and bass player, Mitch Culver, had a lead singer they called "Kid." They were becoming frustrated with his antics and were trying to get rid of him. As Tony put it, "Our lead singer wasn't very good, and all he wanted to do was get drunk. We knew Matt played guitar and heard he was pretty good. As it turned out, he was a better singer too, so we got rid of Kid and brought in Matt."

Matt was ecstatic to finally be in a band that was recording songs and doing shows. Lynda was a little apprehensive because she knew the boys he would be playing with were much older. She was afraid Matt would be negatively influenced by them. I told her not to worry because I'd be at every show, making sure he'd be alright. I had no idea at the time, but Matt was already "negatively influenced," before he became a member of the band. He had been secretly smoking cigarettes and drinking alcohol since he was fourteen!

Matt had visions of being a rock star, and he felt this would be his way of breaking into the music industry. "I want to make music for a living dad," he would often say. He considered getting into a punk band as a stepping-stone to the big time. However, in order to accomplish his goal, he and his band mates Tony and Mitch, would hang out with the counter-culture punks in Bedford.

"We got hooked up with these older guys who were in their mid-twenties. You're gonna do some bad stuff because these kids are older, and they're gonna tell us to fuck off, or do what we do, so we chose to take their crap," Tony admitted to me later. Matt, being the youngest in the group, clearly wanted to fit in. He would be the one to do whatever it took to show he wasn't just an under aged kid. "The older kids liked Matt because he'd go a little further than we would. He would fill in on their sets if one guy went off on a heroin binge or something. He could keep up with them, staying up 'til 4 in the morning, partying with these guys," said Tony.

I began to notice his choice of attire was becoming more radical too. He started wearing a waist-length black leather jacket, loaded with silver studs; he'd spent hours attaching each one. He painted "Subverts" in bold red letters on the sleeve, with ONEWAY SYSTEM, and The Virus painted on the back. He always preferred black skinny jeans, and topping off the look was his prized possessions. A pair of three-inch high platform shoes, glossy black, with three small red and black stars around the sides and back, and a larger red one on the top. At 6'1" in his bare feet, with the shoes Matt stood an imposing 6'4", the tallest, albeit the youngest, member of the band.

Also around this time, I'd overheard him using profanity, cussing like a veteran sailor, when he was around his friends, or talking to them on the phone. I would often tell him to watch his language when he was around the house. "Don't let your mother hear you talking like that!" It seemed like the more I tried to stop his profanity, the more vulgar he'd get.

He did respect my wishes, not using those words around the house. When he didn't think anyone was listening, however, he'd cut loose with some pretty original cuss words. "Fucking shit, motherfucker!" I overheard him say to one of his many phone friends.

Even so, I still thought I'd be able to head off any egregious character changes, as long as I stayed involved with Matt and his music. Besides, dressing differently and using profanity was just teenaged rebellion. He was still doing well in school, so a little bit of contrariness was to be expected at his age. All our other kids did the same thing, in some form or other, so I wasn't too worried about Matt, or his band mates.

What I really wondered was, how did he get into Punk Rock? That form of music is not where you'd expect a young black kid from the suburbs, with a decidedly ethnocentric family, to gravitate towards. We never played it at home… NEVER! So with his obvious talent, why would he waste it on that kind of music? To me, it sounded like the same three chords, played at break-neck speed, and lyrics loaded with profanity, "sung" by screeching, angst-ridden anarchists.

It seemed Matt was just continuing his habit of hanging out with the outsiders. He probably felt skating was a little too childish for him now, and the obvious "progression," as he put it, was to go Punk. Even better, joining a Punk Rock band made him feel he'd finally found his niche. He embraced it whole-heartedly.

As Tony would later say, "The punk scene was a really well-read, self-educated crowd. There were political, religious, social, and cultural ideas going on, and I think Matt picked up on that, and that's what we enjoyed about the scene."

According to Jon Petro, the former lead singer of local punk band Criminal Authority, "Matt didn't just enjoy the life, he lived the life. Matt was the punkest motherfucker you knew!" Being totally oblivious, all I knew about the scene was drinking, violence, and anarchy. Stereotypes all, but that was my perception at the time. I couldn't believe my son would be remotely connected to this way of life. I had no idea what to expect, but I knew Matt wanted to explore this form of music, and no amount of arguing by his parents, or siblings, was going to change his mind.

I justified it by saying, music is music, right? At least he's still playing his guitar and getting a feel of what it's like to be in a band. So, I resigned myself to being supportive, but armed, whenever he had a show.

"Black Matt," as he was affectionately called, absolutely loved the punk scene. He enjoyed being around all the characters that were a part of it. The feeling among the punk community was apparently mutual. "Matt was very welcome in the scene from the start. It was only thought of as unusual because, strictly speaking, he was the only black kid that wanted to be a part of it," Petro said. "He was a true individual in a scene comprised largely of people claiming individuality while conforming to a group mentality. Matt wasn't like that. He was one of the good ones."

As for me, I was waiting to see what this "scene" was all about, and how things would go at one of the Subverts' gigs. I would soon find out because Matt came home very excited a few days later and said, "Dad, we're going to play our first gig this Saturday! Are you gonna come?" Of course I was going, but I asked him where it would be. I was thinking the Agora, or the Grog Shop, or someplace like that. When he said it was going to be at a place called Thunder Alley, I instantly thought, "I'm goin' in strapped!"

CHAPTER 7
THUNDER ALLEY

By definition, the punks of the early 2000s were considered the misfits or outcasts of society, and therefore had their own special community. As former punk band Criminal Authority lead singer Petro so eloquently put it, "The punk scene in every city, and surrounding towns and suburbs, is like a family – very close. Everyone knows everyone. Some people will say it's about politics and angst and all that rubbish, and that is a part of it, but it's mostly about kids who just identify with the counter-culture, whatever that may be. Punks are musicians, artists, poets, activists, as well as the usual lot of jaded nihilists who just like drinking beer, listening to fast music, and having fun."

As I was driving Matt to Thunder Alley for the show, I was thinking only about my son's safety and how crazy this whole thing was to me. Lynda wouldn't go; she was totally against any of it, so it was left to me to bring our son home unharmed. "I've heard about what goes on at those punk rock shows," she said, "so you'd better not let anything happen to Matt." Those words were going through my head as I pulled up to this dilapidated, two-story building at the corner of 30th and Payne Ave., in the heart of the inner city known as the "dirty 30s," or what is now called Cleveland's Chinatown. The place was owned by someone in the punk community, and they allowed punk bands to play there as a sort of underground venue.

There was no signage to let you know this was Thunder Alley, but apparently it was the right place because we saw Tony and Mitch, on the outside of the building, smoking cigarettes. "Hey dude, we've been waiting for you," Tony said to Matt. By now, Matt was so eager to play in front of an audience, he could barely stand still. "Let's do it', he said, and walked into the bar with his guitar, as if it were the most natural thing in the world.

I followed them into the building and could see right away that this was going to be a harrowing experience for me. It was already pretty crowded, and the drinks were flowing freely. I could even smell marijuana, and there was no telling what other kinds of drugs were being abused. The crowd was all spiked hair, shaved heads, black gear, and Doc Martins. You could almost feel the angst in the room, and the alcohol-fueled testosterone levels were exceptionally high.

My first thought was, "What has Matt gotten us into?" Other than Matt's band mates, I saw no familiar faces in the crowd, at least any I could recognize. It was very dark with very little lighting, and the walls were painted black, which made it even harder to see, but I was pretty sure none of Matt's skateboarding friends would be found here… *their* parents wouldn't think of it!

Even though this crowd would normally be called misfits in the society I was familiar with, I was the one feeling like a misfit in this sea of black garments and profanity-laced conversations. Nowhere did I see another black face in the bar, but more alarming to me was I didn't see any form of security either. With all these potential sticks of human dynamite ready to explode at any minute, why wasn't there any security? I was already feeling uncomfortable, but now I was a little frightened, not only for me, but for Matt. I slowly reached up and felt the gun I'd stashed in my inside coat pocket and felt a little better. If anybody came at me or my son, I was perfectly willing to light their asses up. I was ready to go to jail to keep Matt out of harm's way.

After a while, my eyes adjusted to the dim light, and I was able to make out more details in my surroundings. I could see the members of the mostly male all-white crowd were in their late teens or early twenties. The young girls I saw were dressed mostly in black, their lipstick too, but you could tell some of them were probably too young to even be up this late at night; it must have been well past their bedtime. It seemed like everyone was smoking, and the cloud of tobacco and marijuana smoke was so thick in the room, if you inhaled enough of it, you'd either wind up with cancer, or a contact high.

I could tell I was the oldest one in the place and stuck out like a sore thumb. I was dressed like a dad at a soccer game—polo shirt, Dockers, and Nike's. Even the coat I wore had a Shaker Heights Country Club logo prominently displayed on the front. I felt as if the whole crowd was eyeing me suspiciously, and in hindsight, they probably were. Rather than get myself all worked up about the situation, I decided to go to the bar and get myself a beer.

There was another band playing; guitars screeching; drums beating relentlessly, and the lead "singer" was working the mosh pit faithful into a frenzy. I worked my way through the bedlam to the bar. It wasn't really a bar in the common sense, but a huge tub full of beer, and various bottles of whiskey on display on a table next to it. The hulking "bartender" was bald. He must have weighed at least 300 lbs. and was well over six feet tall, with arms that looked as big as tree trunks, sleeve tattoos covering both in their entirety. He looked at me with weary eyes and said, "What'll it be pops?"

"Just a beer, thanks" I said, trying to show I was not a threat, or worse, a cop!

"Two dollars," was all he said, to which I hurriedly paid the man and looked around for a place to sit and watch the show.

I located a dark corner of the room near the stage but far enough from the mosh pit to be safe, and waited for the Subverts to perform. Thankfully, the first band had ended their set, and the sudden quiet was almost painful. It seemed to me as soon as the music stopped, the crowd became dormant, and while the conversations were still profanity-laced, they were somehow more intelligent.

As I was drinking my beer and waiting for the show to start again, hopefully with Matt, a tall, skinny young man, dressed in the ubiquitous black with a spiked Mohawk, sidled over to me and said ominously, "What are you doin' here, pops?" I apparently was right in my assumption that they knew I was the oldest one there;that was the second time tonight I'd been called "pops." Not expecting anyone to talk to me, I was caught a little off guard. I couldn't think of anything clever to say, so I told the truth. "I'm here to see the Subverts. My son plays lead guitar with them."

The punk slowly started to smile and said, "You're Black Matt's dad? Dude, your son is awesome!" I wasn't sure if he was trying to get me to lower my defenses, or if he was sincere, so I simply said, "Come again?" Mohawk was really animated now, tattooed arms flailing around as he spoke. "Dude, your son is probably the best punk guitarist I've ever heard. He's the reason I came."

I was flabbergasted, to say the least. Even more so when he yelled to the group of punks seated next to my table. "Hey, this is Black Matt's old man!" I was immediately surrounded by white boys dressed in black, tattooed arms giving me bear hugs instead of handshakes, with hearty slaps on the back for good measure. "Hey man, what you drinkin'?" said one of the punks. Before I could say I hadn't finished my first beer yet, at least three more beers, and a couple of shots of whiskey, magically appeared on the table in front of me. The Mohawk punk I'd originally met saw me looking at the drinks cautiously and said, "Don't worry pops, just drink what you can. What you don't finish won't get wasted." Then he helped himself to one of the beers on the table, which I was eternally grateful for, and proceeded to help me out.

A young lady in the group was regaling me with stories about the local punk scene. How Matt was rapidly making a name for himself as a true punk guitarist. The stage lights were turned up, and a guy in a tight black t-shirt, and black jeans, with close-cropped hair shouted into the mic. "Alright you assholes! Are you ready for the next band?" Everyone yelled their affirmations, and the announcer said, "Here, for the first time at Thunder Alley, the Subverts!"

The house lights were lowered and everyone got quiet in anticipation of what was to come. Then, the bright spotlight turned on the stage, and I saw my son move to the mic and say in a loud voice, "I hate fuckin' authority," and went into one of their original Subverts tunes, "Authority Sux." I watched as the mosh pit instantly filled with muscular bodies, bumping and smashing mindlessly into one another. The Subverts, specifically Matt, was plowing through his power chords at lightning speed, and to their credit, Tony and Mitch were keeping pace.

The group I'd been sitting with headed to the mosh pit and blended right in with the chaos on the "dance floor." Spiked Mohawk (I never got his name) stayed behind, sitting there watching the commotion and sipping his beer. When I asked why he wasn't joining his buddies in the pit, he said matter-of-factly, "If I went in there and one of those motherfuckers messed up my hair, I'll kill him." Startled at his comment, I looked over at him to see if he was joking, but the look in his eyes told me he was serious.

No longer feeling comfortable, I grabbed my beer, downed one of the shots of whiskey (just to be polite), thanked Mohawk for the drinks, and got away from him. I used the excuse of wanting to get a closer vantage point to better see the band. I found another location that was relatively secluded and sat down to watch Matt play. I never liked punk rock, and to be honest, even the Subverts stuff was not that good. However, what I noticed more than the music was the absolute look of euphoria on Matt's face.

His nystagmus, which he'd had from birth, wouldn't

allow him to see clearly things at a distance, so I don't think he was able to make out facial details in the fast-moving mosh pit. But he was the consummate showman as he worked his way around the stage, hitting those power chords with an alacrity that defied his obvious inebriated state. Yes, I said inebriated. After almost every song, he and his band mates were given beers, which they would guzzle down before going into their next fast-paced jam.

I'd seen enough and was ready to grab Matt by the ear, drag him off that stage and into the safe confines of my car when a serious commotion developed just outside the entrance to the bar. Black-garbed punks began to run outside, spiked haired punks taking swings at skinheads on the way out the door. It seemed like the whole place was turning into a fight club. Since I was sitting away from the door, I was able to see everything going on in the bar. Most of the mosh pit had gone outside, and the group I'd been sitting with earlier were headed that way too. I saw Mohawk coming toward me and reached inside my coat, getting ready to pull out my gun. When he got to my table he said, "Don't go outside, pops. They're stompin' people out there!" and then he ran outside, apparently to join the fray.

"I hope no one messes up his hair. There's going to be a murder out there," I thought,

Incredibly, the Subverts kept on playing to a greatly reduced audience and completed their first set. Afterward,

Matt announced they were going to take a break, and seeing me seated in the corner, he came over, having the presence of mind to leave the beer behind. "Hey dad, what did you think? Isn't this awesome?" he said excitedly. I couldn't believe my baby boy was so calm and seemingly undisturbed by the encroaching danger I knew was imminent.

"Matt, we're gettin' out of here. Get your stuff and let's go! I said. He gave me a look as if to say, "Are you crazy?" and said,

"Don't worry dad. These guys won't hurt us. We're the entertainment. We're taking our break now because when they get through fighting, they'll want to hear some more music. I can't leave. We have another set to play." I couldn't believe what I was hearing. I'm standing here in fear for my life, and my fifteen-year-old son is telling me he has to play some more. Am I the only one that's wondering what's wrong with this picture?? Lynda's words came back to mind: "… you better not let anything happen to Matt." and I said, "Get your stuff, Matt, I'm not leaving you here by yourself."

He gave me a despairing look and said, "Please dad, I promise we can leave after this last set. I'll be totally embarrassed if I have to leave because my dad pulled me off stage."

I was about to insist until I thought about how I'd feel if I couldn't finish a show because of my parents. How I'd probably never be able to live it down. I looked around at the gathering crowd; the fighting must have ended because Mohawk was back at my former table, slamming down a shot of whiskey, hair no worse for the wear. I knew instantly Matt would be the laughing stock of this group for some time to come. "Black Matt had to leave 'cuz his daddy wouldn't let him stay!" or, "Black Matt can't hang with us; we'd have to worry about his daddy kickin' the door in when it gets past dark!"

Reluctantly, I agreed to let him finish the last set, "But we're leaving as soon as it's over," I said sternly. He gave me a hug, said "Thanks dad," and hurried back to the stage. I went over to Mohawk and saw there was still a lone shot of whiskey on the table. "You mind?" I asked as I pointed to the drink. He didn't look up at me, just kept watching the entrance to the bar, and said, "Help yourself, pops." I downed the whiskey in one gulp, enjoying the warmth it generated on the way down my throat.

My nerves settled somewhat; I could hear police sirens getting closer in the distance. As if that sound was some sort of signal, the crowd of punks filed slowly back into the bar. With the exception of a bruised eye here and a bloody lip there, the majority of them showed no signs of "people getting stomped out there," (although I found out later, someone Matt knew actually did get stomped pretty badly). As Matt predicted, the crowd started chanting, "where's the band," and the stage lights dimmed once more.

When the set was finally over, I went looking for Matt. I found him sitting on the side of the stage, talking to a girl with purple hair and black fishnet stockings. "Sorry to interrupt, but it's time to go son," I said. The girl gave him a kiss on the cheek and walked away sheepishly.

"This was the best, dad," Matt said. "I could do this forever!" He packed his guitar and said his goodbyes to his band mates. We then walked the short block to the car, not saying anything on the way.

As I drove home, I looked over to see Matt sound asleep in the passenger seat. He had a little smile on his face, as if he was having an incredibly pleasant dream. I thought back on the little boy I'd taken to guitar lessons a few years ago, and how innocent he looked as he tried to explain to me what *arpeggio* was. I remember thinking he would never be that kid again, now that he'd tasted that intoxicating ambrosia called performing. There would be no turning back for him.

I was happy for him, but worried as well. I'd have to talk to him about the drinking, and yes, the smoking too! (I'd seen him hitting someone's cigarette during the commotion at the bar.) My only wish was that this punk rock phase wouldn't last long, and that I'd get to hear him perform some "real" music in the near future!

CHAPTER 8

Gonzo Life

After the Thunder Alley show, Matt was feeling like he'd finally found his calling. "I told you I'd be good, dad. I'm the lead guitarist in a punk band, and people like how I play!" I didn't have the heart to tell him it doesn't take a genius to play three power chords over and over. I didn't want to curb his enthusiasm. I was just happy to see him happy, but Lynda was more concerned with the crowd he was hanging with.

"He's only fifteen years old. He's playing in these dive bars with people much older than that. They're grown men, for God's sake! Why do you let him do it?" she said, almost in a resigned voice. We'd had this conversation before. I was enjoying watching Matt perform at their shows. Even at such a young age, he had total control of his instrument, and by extension, the audience. The young male punks in the crowd would respond like Pavlov's dogs when Matt would fly into his guitar solos. As soon as they heard the music, they'd rush to the front of the stage and spastically dance around. The young punk girls would look longingly at Matt as he held them enthralled with his guitar and singing.

I tried to justify my leniency. "His grades are still good, and other than an increase in his use of profanity, I don't see why you're so worried. I'm at all of his shows."

"But you're not at all of his *practices!*" She brought up what I had secretly thought myself. When he first started with the Subverts, I was the one who took him to practice. Now, after he'd played a couple of shows, he would have Tony or Mitch pick him up. They wouldn't bring him back home until after midnight sometimes. Lynda hadn't seen Matt smoking cigarettes and drinking beer, but I had. He was wise enough not to do it at home, but I was afraid he would indulge in whatever the rest of the band was doing at their "practices."

Still, I wanted him to continue his band experience (I was still living vicariously through him, I guess). Besides, I was sure he'd grow tired of the punk music, and find another, more "traditional" band to join when he got a little older. "I'll keep a close watch on him, okay?" I said. Lynda just shook her head and walked away.

As it turns out, Lynda was right in her assumptions. While

I naively thought Matt wouldn't do anything more than what I'd witnessed, he was doing exactly what she was afraid of… and more! The Bedford punks were embracing Matt whole-heartedly, and in turn, he would go to extremes to show them he was worthy of their adoration.

"He would be willing to hurt himself a little bit to entertain the group," said his friend, Sarah Solomon, a cute blond with quiet reserve. She was part of the Bedford punk scene when Matt was heavily involved. "He was very outgoing and a little obnoxious sometimes, but I liked him because he was different." Colleen Allison, Sam's girlfriend and Matt's closest female friend, was a bit more specific.

"He would put matches out on his tongue to impress the girls, but that's nothing compared to when he'd ask someone to kick him in the nuts! I even did it once." He'd gotten into letting people kick him in the groin to prove his ability to control pain. "I can't tell you how many times he did that," said Joe Revay, another member of Matt's inner circle. "It never seemed to affect him at all."

With all the rowdiness, drinking, and getting high, the only redeeming quality about the scene was how well read the punks were. Matt loved to talk about everything, and the Bedford punks were his sounding board. Even though the scene was filled with all the vices one could imagine, he could still have intelligent, and stimulating, conversations. Philosophy, individualism, existentialism, and even metaphysics. Subjects

Matt had read about but couldn't discuss with anyone before now because, "Nobody wants to talk with me about that stuff, other than the punks."

Matt's presence with the "Bedford Kids" gave them bragging rights of sorts, since he was one of the very few black kids in the scene. As Tony Furino put it, "Being black in the punk scene made him one in a hundred... and we had him." There apparently were punk factions in different suburbs around Cleveland, the main rivalry for Bedford being the Parma Kids. "We'd come into shows with Black Matt, and everyone would think it was so cool. We had a black punk, and they didn't," said Tony.

It was also during this time that Matt started reading books by Hunter S. Thompson, a troubled but brilliant writer whose caustic wit and acerbic style of writing was heavily influenced by drugs and alcohol. His devil-may-care spirit and unmitigated disdain for authority made him the perfect role model for Matt to emulate.

He started writing constantly in notebooks that he carried around everywhere he went, documenting various conversations, or jotting down words he wanted to find the meaning of later. We didn't know he was secretly drinking and drugging while experimenting with his writing, trying to duplicate the prowess of his hero, Hunter S. Thompson.

Take, for example, Matt's early written observation on what he called our, "toilet society": "I know now our society is so full of shit that it might as well be a fucking toilet. Dishonesty is most likely the root of it all. Ignorance is the seed. What we have now is the tree. But it's not a beautiful tree, no it's not. This is a toilet waiting to be flushed, and a tree ready to be rooted! However, I do not wish to impose my theory on anyone. I will structure my life with my own theory, and live by it. This is my prerogative."

He also began to read books with titles like, Acid Dreams,, by Martin A. Lee and Bruce Shlain, and The Varieties of Psychedelic Experience – The classic guide to the effects of LSD on the human psyche, by Robert Masters and Jean Houston. Matt and his friends even read, The Turner Diaries, written by National Alliance leader, William L. Pierce. This struck me as odd because it was about a white supremacist guerilla army, but Matt didn't seem to think it was anything more than intellectual enlightenment. "Punks aren't racists, dad; they wouldn't let me be a part of the scene if they were," he said, which did nothing to ease my ever increasing concerns.

In keeping with his newfound punk/rocker identity, Matt was getting more attention from the young ladies. Lynda and I had given Matt the "sex talk" when he first joined the band, but he didn't want to hear it at the time. "Come on mom, do we have to talk about this now? This is embarrassing!" It seems his protestations were just an act because he'd already had sex for the first time a couple of years before, at the age of thirteen. "He lost his virginity to a girl named Janine back in

2000," said his best friend Sam. "Matt had no problem talking to the girls, even back then."

As Criminal Authority's Petro remembered, "Everyone in the scene liked Matt. The girls really loved him. They all wanted to see the "Green Mile." He'd apparently taken to calling his penis that, and had no qualms about showing it off.

As one of the girls would tell me later, "Matt was well-endowed, and proud of it. He got me with the personal groomer story, and I'm like, 'really, you do that? Can I see?' He whips it out, and sure enough, he was clean-shaven down there." She continued, "He had no problem in the package department, and you wouldn't expect it from someone so skinny!"

At Heskett Middle School where he was a student, he was getting a reputation as a "bad-ass" among his classmates. He got busted for selling marijuana with one of his Bedford friends during school hours. The ensuing three-day suspension for the offense was a far cry from the expulsion he was in danger of getting. It took much pleading from me, and crying from his mother, to persuade the principal to give him another chance.

Matt was growing up fast, and it seemed there was nothing we could do about it. In Lynda's and my defense, he took advantage of the fact we both worked full time and couldn't monitor him as closely as we would have liked. He was a "latch key kid," and would come home from school, do his homework, and be gone before we got there. He would always call to let us know he was at band practice, and because he hadn't gotten into any more trouble at school, we had no reason to doubt him.

Matt's involvement with the Subverts lasted a couple of years, until Tony Furino decided he was going to college and didn't want to be in a punk band anymore. Matt and Mitch Culver continued hanging out with the Bedford punks, and specifically, with Jon Petro, the leader of Criminal Authority. Petro shared a huge house in Walton Hills with his mother, and since she spent most of her time in Finley, Ohio, Jon was given full reign. There was no limit to what Matt was able to do at the house. At sixteen, he was usually the youngest person in the place, but he was able to consume as much beer, or smoke as much marijuana as any of the older kids— sometimes more.

I even asked him once why he was still hanging out with that crowd now that the Subverts had broken up. He was adamant when he said, "Dad, I have a chance to play with Criminal Authority, but I have to be around them so I can learn their music. Once I do, they'll let me play in some of their shows." I knew Criminal Authority was the local punk band in Bedford. They had a loyal following and were local celebrities in the punk scene. Matt was one of their biggest fans; he'd acquired a CD from the group and played it incessantly, to the chagrin of Lynda's and my ears. Matt thought being invited to play with Criminal Authority was the ultimate compliment. Still, wanting him to get better with his guitar (although I was skeptical that would happen with these guys), I reluctantly agreed to let him continue practicing with them.

I soon regretted my decision. One night, I got a call from the Walton Hills police. The officer informed me that Matt was at their station after being picked up, with other underage kids, at the Petro house. Apparently, there was an underage girl there whose parents had called up to say she was at the house with a bunch of grown men. She was only sixteen years old but rebellious, and they knew she'd hung out at Jon's house in the past. The parents wanted the police to go there and get their daughter, which they did, and in the process, arrested everybody under the age of eighteen.

Tony Furino happened to be there at the time too. He'd just returned from college and was interested in starting another band with Matt, but he wanted to go in another direction, leaving punk music behind. "Me and Matt were talking about starting a blues band, and he wanted to bring Mitch in, but I kinda wanted to get out of the scene then," he said. Allegedly, Mitch's girlfriend was the underage girl the cops were looking for, thus the reason for them being arrested. "I almost got charged with kidnapping that night," Tony said. "Me and Matt were just there trying to get a band together, but after that, I totally washed my hands of the whole thing."

I picked Matt up at the Walton Hills station, with a warning from the police to not let him near that house again. "That's not a place you want your son," the officer told me, and I totally agreed. I was putting a stop to Matt's punk affiliation, once and for all. "Matt, that's the last time you're going over there, and I don't care if it means you won't be playing with Criminal Authority."

He just said "okay" and fell silent on the drive home.

Even though he didn't say anything, I knew this was not going to be the last time I'd have to be concerned with Matt and his "involvements." He was much too interested in experiencing life, and this was just a small bump in the road, to be rolled over, and forgotten.

CHAPTER 9

The Point of Saturation

There is a point inside of everyone. This is the point of ignition for some.
When that fuse runs short, whatever you have will depend on if you
decide to color me good or bad.
I am not insane, no, I am not a crazy man. Indeed, I maintain my sanity
the best way I can.
But do not forget that every man has a device. And that device lies in his
will to fight.
Only when a boy grows into maturation, only then will he understand
the point of saturation.
When the blood boils into a cold blue, only then will he be left with
nothing else to do.
-The Point of Saturation, poem by Matthew Green-

The enthusiasm Matt had shown for the punk scene, and the music he played for that crowd, would turn out to be the least of my worries. Lynda and I were starting to notice a distinct change in his behavior in 2002, when he was fifteen. He would say we were stressing him out, and ran away from home twice, causing his mother and I to panic and call the police. Both times, one of his friends knew where he was and talked him into coming back home.

School was apparently stressing him out too because his teachers at the local high school would call us to say Matt was being disruptive in class. He was making the other students uncomfortable, and even frightening them. "He's very scary sometimes, Mr. Green," one of them told me when I came to pick him up for one of his many suspensions.

His acting out concerned us enough to seek a psychologist. Dr. Raymond Hastings was a clinical psychologist we found through the Cleveland Clinic. 'This guy will get Matt straightened out,' I naively thought. 'He's a professional. He'll know what to do to get Matt back." I was being presented with something I'd never been exposed to before. I knew there were instances of mental illness in my family (my mother and my deceased sister come to mind), but I wasn't too worried about Matt in that way. I felt he was intelligent enough to understand what he would need to do in order to get better. After all, wasn't he the one with the high I.Q.?

After a few sessions, Hastings told me Matt seemed to be going through a form of adolescent psychosis, a common occurrence at his age, but treatable with the right medication, and talk therapy.

Psychosis? According to Webster's definition, psychosis is: "a mental disorder . . . that indicates impaired contact with reality." I thought back on Matt's recent behavior. I knew what the teachers had told me, but what I'd witnessed personally made me wonder if the doctor was right.

For a few days prior to his most recent suspension from school, Matt had been talking to Lynda and I about his "obligation to enlighten" the youth of this country to his way of thinking. "I need to speak with the youth and get them to rise up against authority," he'd say.

"And what are they going to do once you get them to 'rise up?'" I'd asked him.

"We could make our own community and live without parental interference!",was his emphatic response.

He started talking about death and suicide around this time too, and saying how he could get people to kill for him,if he wanted. I wasn't sure if this was just the nihilist talk of his punk scene fantasies, or if he was actually thinking of pursuing this outrageous plan. "Okay Matt, send 'em over here first, so you can see if they're any good. If they get by me, you've got some real killers."

He gazed at me as if to say, 'don't be silly,' and just said matter-of-factly, "Why would I send them to sudden death?" I guess he wasn't that disconnected from reality. Either way, it was disturbing to hear him talk like this. Lynda, especially, was getting worried.

"We've got to get Matt some help," she'd say, and that's when Dr. Hastings became involved.

For a year, Matt's sessions with the doctor seemed to help. His antics in school either stopped, or he wasn't as disruptive, because the frequent calls from his teachers came less and less. His grandiose talk of "leading the youth" wasn't mentioned again, but every now and then he'd say something that would let us know it was still on his mind. "The youth of today are so blind," he'd say to no one in particular.

Another event causing stress in Matt's life around this time was his maternal grandfather, Charles Fields, who was very ill and dying from cancer. He'd worked for more than twenty years at the Ford Stamping Plant in Walton Hills, making brake linings. The apparent inhalation of the asbestos fibers in the air over the years had taken its toll. He was also a heavy smoker during that time, which probably didn't help either.

From a very young age, Matt looked to Charles as his musical guru. "Beaver," as Charles was affectionately called by his contemporaries, was a trumpet player and singer for several jazz bands during the 60s and 70s. He still performed regularly, until his illness prevented him from continuing.

He would often bring Matt sheet music to practice and would drop by a few days later to see how well he'd progressed. Charles would challenge Matt to mimic what he heard on records, with his guitar, the same notes played by trumpeters Herb Alpert and Al Hirt. Matt did it, almost to perfection, for which Charles give him a big hug and made a big deal about how good his grandson was. Matt loved his grandfather immensely and was quite distressed when he learned his mentor was dying.

Not only that, Matt's best friend, Sam Sizemore, was about to move to Spain. His mother had joined the Air Force and was being deployed to that country. "Dad, Sam's moving to Spain with his mother. I'm never gonna be able to find someone I can play music with now," he complained. Both of his musical allies would be unavailable to him, the thought of which caused Matt to abandon his guitar and become more rebellious around the house.

That's when his misbehaving in school started up again. In May of 2003, he was suspended for a third time since the beginning of the fall semester. He was still going to his therapy sessions with Hastings, but that alone was no longer helping as much as it once had.

Dr. Hastings told me after one of their sessions, "You might want to contact a psychiatrist for Matt, so he can get medication. I can give you a recommendation if you like." I was still in denial about Matt's mental state, so I respectfully declined his offer.

"That's okay, doc," I said. "I don't think we're at that point yet." Little did I know, "that point" would come in less than a month.

On May 27, 2003, after a long courageous fight, Charles "Beaver" Fields lost his battle with cancer and passed away. Matt was devastated. He tried not to let it show; he'd always been able to hide his feelings, but we could tell he wasn't his usual self. He sought refuge from his depression in the punk community he so loved, but drugs had pretty much decimated the scene. "The heroin epidemic had the punk scene by the throat," said Criminal Authority's Petro. "Hell, the whole city was getting high!"

Matt even joined the Criminal Authority band, trying to alleviate his sorrow. According to Richie Kray, another member of the band, "We stole him from the Subverts. He was, by far, the best guitar player we'd ever worked with. Unfortunately, the band kind of dissolved a few months after he joined." The reason the band broke up was heroin. As Petro would say candidly, "Looking back, I feel pretty bad for the rest of our band. They were mostly straight, but a couple of us wouldn't even strap on a guitar until we had a good fix. That was the beginning of the end of the band."

This was when Matt began self-medicating in earnest and went from occasionally smoking marijuana to indulging in more extreme forms of drug use. His natural curiosity led him to try cocaine, pharmaceutical acid, mushrooms, and even the one drug his friends were afraid he might try, and like... heroin.

He got started on that with a young lady I'll call "Lilly." She was four years older and already deeply ensconced in the heroin spider web. She and Matt would hang out and get high on several occasions. "I felt really bad about getting him started," she said in an email to me years later. All this was going on unbeknownst to his mother and I (Matt had become intensely private), but his close friends were aware. They voiced their disapproval to him, but out of loyalty, or more likely Matt's coercions, said nothing.

His grandfather's funeral was the tipping point. All during the memorial service, he was agitated and restless. He couldn't seem to keep still for more than a minute or two. He'd get up and leave the sanctuary only to return a little while later, wide-eyed and fidgety. When the pastor asked for acknowledgements, Matt got up and strode to the podium. He began by saying how much his grandfather meant to him, and how he could always count on his support. For the first couple of minutes, everything seemed normal. He spoke quite eloquently as he described how Charles helped him learn to play his guitar, using the notes from his trumpet as a guide.

Then, a strange look came into Matt's eyes, and he started looking up at the ceiling of the church, as if he were expecting to see something come crashing right through the roof. That's when he began talking disjointedly, and continuously, about any and everything, none of which had anything to do with the proceedings. I thought, at first, he was just handling his grandfather's death in his own unique way, but it turned out he was exhibiting full-blown psychosis. I walked up to the podium and gently coaxed him back to his seat, slightly embarrassed, but determined, more than ever to get Matt the help he needed.

Two days after the funeral, Matt was hospitalized for the first time. He'd come home from school, cursing loudly and pacing around the house like a caged animal. Dr. Hastings told us to take him to Cleveland Clinic because they had a psychiatric ward especially for adolescents. There, he could get the treatment he needed immediately. Lynda and I were torn because we loved our son so much, but knew he had to have the help we couldn't provide.

Matt was kept for a week before he was discharged, with instructions to continue follow-up treatment with his personal psychiatrist. As I said earlier, I hadn't taken his psychologist up on his offer to recommend a child psychiatrist, but now I was forced to. Matt had to have prescriptions for the medications he needed to maintain his mental balance, and I was going to make sure he got it.

Through Dr. Hastings, we found Dr. Terry Miller, Ph.D. She was a delightful woman with a pleasant personality who seemed to genuinely care about Matt's well-being. After having a few sessions with Matt, she officially diagnosed him as having bipolar affected disorder, one common with adolescents, and gave us prescriptions for the medications he would need. She said as long as he took the meds as instructed and continued therapy with Dr. Hastings, he could conceivably be taken off the medication in a few years. Because he was only sixteen years old, she felt he could possibly be symptom-free by his early twenties, "But he has to take the meds, consistently, every day," she warned.

Under her and Hastings' care, Matt was able to keep his behavior under control, and his erratic mood swings were almost non-existent. He was doing very well in school, and luckily, his grades didn't suffer too much while he was hospitalized. Everything seemed to be back to normal, or so we thought, until Lynda came to me with a revelation.

"Matt hasn't been taking his medication," she said.

"What are you talking about?" I asked incredulously.

"I was cleaning out his room, and I found a stash of pills under his bed. They're the pills he's supposed to have been taking!" She was almost beside herself as she told me there must have been a months-worth of pills there.

When I confronted Matt about our find, he simply said, "I feel much better, so I stopped taking them a while ago. I told Dr. Hastings, but Dr. Miller doesn't know."

I was livid! I had to admit, I hadn't seen any change in his behavior, but that didn't mean he wasn't on the precipice of another breakdown. I knew that without the medication he would eventually have a relapse, and with the amount of pills we were now aware he hadn't taken, that could be sooner rather than later. "Matt, you have to take your meds. Not taking them is out of the question!", I admonished.

"But I don't need them anymore", he said, "I feel much better."

Luckily, it was the same day he was scheduled to see

Dr. Miller, so I said, "If the doctor says you don't need them anymore, I'll go along with it, but if she says otherwise, you're going to continue taking the meds. Agreed?" He said something unintelligible, but I was pretty sure the doctor would change his mind.

When we got to her office, I told her Matt hadn't been taking his medication regularly. I also told her about the stash of pills my wife had found under his bed. She didn't look as surprised as I thought she should. She only asked Matt to come with her into a private room so they could talk. About thirty minutes later, she came out and asked Lynda and I to join them in the room. When I entered, I looked over at Matt slouching in his chair. He had a look of stubborn determination on his face. I'd seen this look before, when I'd asked him to cut the grass or shovel snow and he didn't want to do it.

"Mr. and Mrs. Green, I've discussed with your son the importance of taking his medication daily. Of how difficult it can be to regulate his illness every time he relapses." She continued, "However, he seems to think he doesn't need the meds anymore because he's feeling better. I've seen this before. Once a patient starts feeling better because of the medication, they decide to stop, erroneously believing they no longer need it. He's still saying he refuses to take his meds."

I turned to Matt and said, "I thought we agreed to go by what the doctor says."

He gave me a smirk and said, "You agreed, I didn't." I

wanted to slap him upside the head, but I refrained, since I was in front of witnesses.

"You will take your medicine, whether you want to or not!" I said, hoping he could hear the threat in my voice.

He just shrugged his shoulders and said, "No, I'm not. I know better than any of you how I feel, and I don't need any more medicine."

I decided not to argue with him about it and directed my next words to the doctor. "If he doesn't take his meds anymore, what will happen?"

She said, "Since we don't know how long he's been off his meds, and he won't tell me, I think it's plausible to expect him to have a relapse very soon. Each time that happens, it becomes harder to regulate him because of the need for stronger dosages." Then she said something that would resonate with me for the rest of Matt's life. "If he continues to refuse to take his medication as he should, I'm afraid all I can do is be here to help you pick up the pieces."

We left her office without getting any assurances from Matt, but I knew this was the beginning of a battle of wills. His against mine, for better or worse, until one of us gave up. I was determined not to let it be me.

CHAPTER 10

The Gypsy Gibsons

I've seen and done so much with these two eyes of mine, and though they don't see well, I can see your eyes cry.
-Lyrics from "Heart of Gold" by Matt Green-

PART 1

A t sixteen years old, Matt had seen and done things some twice his age hadn't done... or more precisely, would never do.

At this moment, he was sitting on a bench in front of Marymount Hospital lighting a cigarette. He'd just spent the past seven days as a "guest" in Marymount's Psychiatric Ward, the result of not taking his mood stabilizing meds for more than a month.

With the decline of Bedford's punk scene, the death of his grandfather, his best friend Sam about to leave for Spain, and the kids at school badgering him, 2003 was turning out to be a tumultuous year for Matt. The anxiety he felt was overwhelming him, and he didn't know how to channel his frustrations. "I have to make sense of this chaotic plethora of intangible miscellany I call, my mind," he wrote in one of his many notebooks.

He knew he'd been acting more rebellious toward his parents lately. He just couldn't find it within himself to care. He would drive them nuts with his lack of effort while half doing chores around the house, the same chores he'd always done since he lived there. Sometimes, he would flat out refuse to do anything they asked at all, no matter how mundane. He'd start feeling really good, and wasn't about to let vacuuming the carpet, or cutting the grass, spoil it.

He smiled to himself as he thought of how easily he could manipulate them.

His father thought Matt's sojourn into the punk life, at such a young age, was the main reason for his change in attitude. His mother was more specific. She thought it was the punk music that was the culprit. Both theories were partly true, but that wasn't the reason he was smiling.

Matt knew it was because he wasn't getting much sleep, and they had no clue. His mind was racing all the time now, and no matter what he did, he couldn't make himself tired enough to go to sleep. He'd be up for hours during the night, running up and down the stairs, or pacing the hall outside his parent's bedroom door. He knew he woke them because his dad would complain. "Matt, please go back to bed. We're trying to sleep in here!" He'd have to be more careful. To them, his not sleeping was a sure sign of an imminent manic episode. He would have to get better at covering up his insomnia.

He'd already been suspended from school five times, and hospitalized twice for that very reason, this semester alone. Luckily, his unit principal was very understanding and allowed his parents to bring Matt the lessons he missed while in treatment. "I don't want him to get left behind," she'd said.

This time, his sleepless nights had gone on for more than two weeks, causing him to be more and more manic, acting in bizarre ways. The last straw was when his father came home from work and found him sitting on the front porch in his underwear. He was waving a large American flag with one hand and was using his other to toss slices of lunch meat to his dog, Onyx. Onyx was a huge, black Great Dane who stood a full six feet when on his hind legs. He was tied to the porch railing, eagerly waiting for his master to throw him another slice of the most delicious meat he'd ever tasted. For some reason, Matt couldn't stop saying, "God bless America!" at the top of his voice, over and over again. That's how he ended up in Marymount.

He had to admit, he was feeling better now; his mind was as clear as it had ever been. But the mood stabilizing drug's side effects made him feel lethargic. He was aware of the need to continue taking the medicine, so he decided to make the best of the situation.

PART 2

When he came home from the hospital, I noticed Matt wasn't as outgoing as he used to be. I also noticed a change in his routine when he was around the house. He used to come in, go straight to his room, and within a few minutes he'd be playing his guitar, the sounds of his acoustic filling the house. Now, he would only walk around as if in a daze, barely talking to us, and mostly sleeping the day away. He hadn't played for two months since his grandfather died, his guitar sitting abandoned in its case. When I asked him if he was feeling alright, he'd just say, "I've been pretty tired lately. I need more sleep."

I was afraid he was going into a depression, and I mentioned this to Lynda, who suggested I bring it up with his psychologist at his next session. However, since he'd been home, Matt had become secretive and intensely private. He didn't want us to get involved with his aftercare or outpatient treatment. "I can handle my own appointments. I'm the one going through this, so let me handle it." Because he was still a minor, I knew I could contact his doctor when necessary, but I wanted to see if Matt would hold up his end of the bargain.

To his credit, he did keep his appointments, and took his meds as prescribed every day. His mood swings were being managed, but the medication wasn't alleviating the depression he seemed to be in. Lynda and I agreed we should bring it up with Matt's psychiatrist at his next visit. Privacy be damned!

One warm afternoon in August of that year, I'd spent the better part of the day doing yard work. I'd just finished cutting the backyard lawn and killed the mower engine. I usually enjoy the immediate silence of nature, once the ear-numbing decibels of the engine dies and the only real sound you hear is the chirping of the birds. But this particular day I didn't hear the birds. What I heard brought a smile to my face and joy to my heart. I could hear Matt playing his guitar through the open window of his bedroom at the back of the house.

I stopped what I'd been doing, yard work, a thing of the past, and sat in our yard swing slowly rocking to the rhythm of the music he was playing. As I listened closer, I could hear him singing softly in time to his playing. I was overjoyed! After a long hiatus, Matt was actually back to doing what I knew he loved… his music. I felt compelled to go to his room to see what other surprises I'd find once I was able to see him face to face. Would there be that glow in his eyes that comes when he figures out a difficult chord progression? Would his melancholy mood finally be eliminated?

I didn't want to be the reason he'd stop playing if he was interrupted. It had been so long since I'd heard him say more than a few mumbled words before heading to his room to sleep. However, my paternal instincts kicked in, and I realized it was only right that I go up and check on him. After all, since Lynda wasn't home at the time, I felt it was my duty to give her a full report on how her son was doing. She had been worried about his well-being even more than I had.

I quietly climbed the stairs and walked the short hallway to the closed door of his room. His playing got louder as I slowly pushed open the bedroom door. He was sitting on his bed, not aware I had just come into his room. I could see his eyes were closed, totally absorbed in the music he was playing, as he strummed an unfamiliar, but pleasant melody on his guitar. I stood in the doorway, happily listening to Matt play, with my eyes closed, when the music suddenly stopped. He must have felt someone else was in the room because when I opened my eyes, he was staring at me with a slight grin on his face.

"Well, what do you think dad?" was all he said. I was expecting him to be a little angry that I'd invaded his privacy, so I was taken aback when he stood up and came over to give me a big hug! "Dad, I feel like playing again, isn't that great?" he said.

"That is great, son. When did you get the urge to play again?" He didn't answer my query. He just picked up a notebook and handed it to me,.

"I've got over ten songs already written, and I'm working on some more," he said. "What you just heard was one I call, 'Feeling A Feeling.' I wasn't sleeping all the time I was in my room. I was busy writing songs."

I leafed through his notebook and saw he had indeed written several pages of lyrics. I asked him if he had the music to go with all those lyrics, and he said, "I can hear it in my head, but I haven't quite gotten to where I'm ready to play them yet. I need a band to bring these songs to life."

My first thought was, 'here we go again. Another punk band,' but all I said was, "So where are you going to get band members from?"

He gave me a big smile and said, "I've already been working on that. I've even got a name for the band." He didn't wait for me to ask when he said proudly, "The Gypsy Gibsons."

Just when I thought he was going to crash and burn into the depths of depression, he had been secretly planning to form a new band of his own making. Lynda would be thrilled to know her son was coming back around. I asked him to play, "Feeling a Feeling" for me again, and he didn't hesitate. He picked up his guitar, and once again I was able to see the joy on his face and the proud look of accomplishment as he played and sang his song.

PART 3

By the fall of 2003, Matt was obsessed with recording his songs and getting his band together. His first recruit was Jesse Carter, a high school friend Matt had played with at the school talent show, and who happened to have a makeshift recording studio at his house. "I would just record the drum track, and he would go in the recording closet and play all the other instruments, track by track," said Jesse. "It was time-consuming, but we didn't realize it at the time because we were having fun," he continued.

Matt would enlist his good friend, Eric Harms, who played bass and whose house Matt considered his second home, to be the next member of the band. Another long-time friend, Joe Revay, whom Matt had taught to play guitar, would round out the Gypsy Gibsons' membership. They practiced constantly at Eric's house, sometimes cutting class to go there since it was a short walk from the school. "Matt just had it. He was a natural" said Eric's father, John Slawinski. "He was here all the time, practicing with Joe and Eric, and he was even a decent drummer. Matt could do anything with music."

After practicing a few months, the Gypsy Gibsons were ready to be the entertainment for our 2003 Halloween party. "I remember we were stoked when Matt told us we were playing his parents party. We were so nervous, but after we saw the people liked us, we started relaxing and playing even better," said Joe Revay. That was also the first time we'd seen him playing drums, and it surprised our whole family! Lynda and I were so proud of them, and our guests all seemed to enjoy their playing. It looked like our concerns about Matt were temporarily put to the back burner. He had been in compliance with his meds and was getting sleep. I knew how absorbed he could be with his music, and the Gypsy Gibsons would be his primary focus for the foreseeable future. Since this was Matt's "baby," Joe, Eric, and Jesse would have to have the patience of Job when it came to practice. Matt could be relentless when it came to getting the sound exactly the way he wanted it.

For the next couple of years, Matt and the Gypsy Gibsons practiced long hours, perfecting their sound, and recording the music he'd written, resulting in a five song CD. Matt's enthusiasm rubbed off on Jesse, Eric, and Joe, and they put themselves wholeheartedly into the project. Matt's dream of forming his own band had finally come to fruition! They were ready to play some gigs.

"I remember, after one of our late practices, we loaded up my car with all our equipment and rode around looking for a place to play," Jesse would say later. They drove around to different bars, asking to play, for free, but they were told they were too young. "You have to be twenty-one to play here," one bar owner said.

Finally, they ended up at the Winchester in Lakewood. They brazenly walked into the bar, and Matt told the bartender, "We just want to set up and play here tonight." Apparently impressed with their temerity, the bartender gave them permission, and they set up to play. "We played about four or five songs and we got a good response." From then on, the Gypsy Gibsons were on their way, and Matt was the undisputed leader of the band.

CHAPTER 11

Rise and Fall

By the time Matt was a senior in high school, the Gypsy Gibsons were booking shows and had recorded a five-song CD of Matt's original music. Their practices were grueling because of Matt's insistence on getting the songs exactly the way he wanted them to sound. He and Jesse had worked for over a year, painstakingly putting the tracks together for the CD they planned to eventually sell at their shows.

During this time, Matt was most prolific, writing lyrics and music to over fifteen songs. He would stay up long into the night, working on the songs he'd bring to his band at their next practice. Seeing him so involved with his music lulled me into complacency. It had been almost a year since he'd last been hospitalized, so my usual habit of keeping up with his actions wasn't as keen. The only clue was when he became more argumentative.

Lynda and I would find ourselves justifying to him the reasons we still wanted him to do his share of the work around the house. "Matt, will you please take the dog out. Don't make him wait too long," I'd say to him.

"Why is it so important I do it now?" he'd ask, and a long discussion would ensue, usually with me ending up doing it myself. His ego seemed to be on steroids. He couldn't get enough of telling us how good he was as a musician. "My talent is the reason I've got my own band, and my music is going to make me a lot of money one day!" he told me once.

I just thought he was feeling the testosterone rush of going from a pimple-faced adolescent into a guitar playing "rock star" and having the young ladies start to take notice. He was tall and slim, with a good amount of facial hair forming the beginnings of a pretty impressive beard. He was supremely confident around the ladies and was not afraid to strike up a conversation with the prettiest girl in the room. "He didn't care if it was Halle Berry; he would go right up and talk to her," said Joe Revay. He had natural charisma, and a quick wit that drew people to him in a crowd.

Did I mention he'd moved out of the house too? Two days before his eighteenth birthday, he told his mother he couldn't follow our rules anymore, so he was going to move in with his band mate, Jesse Carter. Lynda was taken totally by surprise, but also furious that Matt would be so bold as to leave the house before he graduated from high school! She immediately called me at work to inform me of Matt's decision. After calming her down enough to listen, I told her to let him go. "Lynda, he's been doing his own thing for a long time, so wanting to leave shouldn't be too surprising."

She was still the protective mother hen over her "baby" and wouldn't hear of it. "No! He's not leaving this house!" She said she was going to call John and Danielle to try and help her keep him there, but I knew that would only escalate into possible violence.

I finally said, "Let him go, Lynda. I don't want anybody to get in trouble because Matt's made up his mind to leave. He's just a couple of days from being eighteen, so legally, we can't stop him anyway."

She let him go, but as I found out later, she had some choice words not only for Matt, but Jesse too. According to her, he was being disrespectful to her, and she really got mad when she heard Jesse tell Matt, "Hurry up and get your stuff so I can get you the hell away from here!"

Lynda and I didn't know it at the time, but Matt had been sporadic about taking his medication. He had mentioned in passing that the medicine made him feel sluggish. He felt his "creative flow" was being adversely affected by "the beans," as he called them. "Sometimes, I wish I didn't have to take medicine," he complained one day. "It makes me feel like I'm a zombie! I can't play my music the way I want 'cause my fingers move too slow on that stuff!"

We'd see him staying up late at night, working relentlessly on whatever music he was composing, but we didn't think too much of it. We thought he was taking his meds as prescribed, and he was making his appointments with Dr. Hastings. We thought his enthusiasm for his band, and the minor local success they were having, was the reason for his grandiose ideas about how far they would go. "We're gonna be the biggest thing from northeast Ohio since the Black Keys," he'd exclaim. "You just wait and see!"

Matt had been under the doctor's care for bipolar disorder for two years and was doing very well with managing his needed regimen. However, he had gotten pretty good at covering up any mood swings he may have been having. Neither Lynda nor I could tell any difference in his demeanor. In hindsight, I think he figured out just how much of the meds he needed to take in order to keep us from thinking something was wrong. We had learned to look for certain signs of behavior that were indicators of another manic episode.

Unfortunately for Matt, taking the medication sometimes, instead of daily, could only be covered up so long. It was during this time when he became to his friends, "a small-dose kind of guy." As his friend Melissa Deal would say, "Matt could be so intense (when he was manic) … about everything, and no one could figure out what caused that reaction in him."

Three months after leaving home, and after 48 hours with no sleep, Matt was on the verge of another manic episode. He went to an apartment complex at 216 Center Street in Bedford, just a few blocks from his parents' home. He'd met someone at the library who'd told him he lived there and for Matt to come by and visit sometime. The only problem was he never told Matt what his name was, or what apartment number he lived in.

To Matt, this didn't seem like an impossible hurdle for him to negotiate. 'I know what he looks like, and I'll just ring all the doorbells at the apartment until he comes down and answers.' he thought. In his state of mind, made fuzzier due to lack of sleep, this seemed to be an excellent idea! He walked from the house he shared with Jesse to the apartment complex a mile away and proceeded to do just that. He started ringing all the residents' buzzers and demanded to be let in when they'd get on the intercom. "Who is it?", came one male voice from the tiny speaker.

"It's Matt. Buzz me in," said Matt.

"Matt who?" the obvious follow up question.

"Matt Green. We met at the library a couple days ago," he said.

"I don't know any Matt Green. You have the wrong apartment."

That went on several more times, with other residents,

until someone actually buzzed him in. He didn't know if it was the friend he was looking for, but he thought whoever did it would come down to see who it was. It might be him. He walked boldly to one of the comfortable looking couches arranged around a large square coffee table and sat down heavily. He knew he should be tired from all the sleep he'd missed, but he wasn't tired at all! He felt like he could stay up for another 24 hours if he wanted to. Maybe his friend would come down to get him and have some weed to smoke. That would be great!

However, Matt's incessant ringing of the door buzzers had caused a concerned (frightened?) resident to call the apartment manager to investigate. Matt casually looked over as the manager came toward him. The man couldn't have been more than a few inches over five feet tall, and had a build almost as wide as he was tall. Matt chuckled as he thought of what his father would call this dude. "Now that's what you'd call a 'sidewalk semi,' his dad would say with his dry humor.

Five-by-five strode up to Matt, who was still seated on the lobby couch. "Sir, who are you here to see?" He tried to sound authoritative, but Matt could hear a little tremble in his voice.

"I'm here to see a friend. He already buzzed me in. I'm just waiting for him to come down," Matt said.

"What is your friend's name?" the manager asked, still trying to keep control of the situation. By now, Matt had had enough. He stood up to his full six-foot, one-inch height, and looked down on Mr. Five-By-Five with his eyes moving wildly side to side, in his signature, intimidating stare.

"I don't have to tell you anything. My friend buzzed me in, and I'm going to wait on him until he comes down," he said in a voice just above a whisper. Because Matt hadn't raised his voice, and the disturbing way his eyes moved, made the manager want to get away from this guy as quickly as possible. 'They're not paying me to be security,' he thought, and did a perfect military about face, and quick-stepped back to his apartment, yelling over his shoulder, "I'm calling the police!"

The mania was almost full blown now, and Matt was feeling invincible. He didn't care if the cops came. By the time they got there, his friend would have already come down for him, and the flatfoots wouldn't even know where he was. 'Damn, I'm smart!' The exuberance he felt in this near-manic state was almost annoying in its intensity. He started getting more agitated. "Go ahead and call. I'm still not leaving," he yelled at the manager's closing door.

Matt felt perfectly justified in being there. The high he was feeling was invigorating and energizing. He was feeling more vital than he had in months, and he knew it was because he'd stopped taking his meds. He was taking them here and there, just to maintain some semblance of a routine around his parents. However, just two days before his 18th birthday, he had moved out of his parent's house and in with band mate,

Jesse Carter. Once there, his self-medication began in earnest, and his "routine" came to a halt. Three months, later he was in this apartment complex, "looking for a friend."

He sat back down on the lobby couch and pulled out a cigarette. He was aware there was no smoking allowed in the building, but in his present frame of mind, he didn't care. He popped the cigarette between his lips and pulled out a Zippo lighter from his jeans pocket. Without hesitation, he fired up. He inhaled deeply, enjoying the temporary calming effect the tobacco had on his psyche. He leaned back on the couch, closed his eyes, and exhaled, fully clearing his lungs before opening his eyes. When he did, he saw a Bedford police cruiser pulling up in front of the complex.

Matt continued smoking and watched as Mr. Five-by-Five escorted two Bedford police officers into the lobby. The two cops looked to Matt as if they were an odd couple. The first one was tall, about an inch taller than Matt, and still had the baby-face look of a high school kid. He stood ramrod straight and stared at Matt with unblinking eyes. His partner was older, with a stocky build. He had to look up at Matt to talk to him, but he appeared to be the one in charge.

"Stand up and put out that cigarette," he ordered. Matt did as he was told, stubbing out the butt with his fingers, and standing up slowly. "What's your name?'" short cop asked.

"Matthew Green." he was talking to short cop but was glancing over at the tall one. He hadn't said a word so far, but Matt could see the muscles under his uniform shirt were tense. "Do you have any identification?" he continued. Matt slowly reached into his back pocket for his wallet, and a slight movement where Tall Cop was standing caught his attention. Did he just reach for his gun? Short Cop must have seen Matt's reaction and stepped between the two of them. "Please hand me your I.D.," he said and held out his hand. This seemed to calm Matt down, and he gave him his credentials.

"We've been called here because the manager says you refuse to leave the premises." He handed Matt back his I.D. Matt looked beyond the two cops and saw the manager grinning from ear to ear but standing a safe distance behind them.

"I have a friend who lives here. I came to visit him but I didn't have his apartment number, so I hit all the buzzers hoping to get some help." He pointed at the manager and said, "That guy wouldn't help me. All he did was keep telling me to leave."

"What's your friend's name?"

"I'm don't know for sure, I only met him once, but he told me he lives here," which made perfect sense to Matt.

"Listen Matt, if you don't know who it is your visiting, and you don't know the apartment number, you have to leave right now."

"I'm not leaving until I see my friend." Matt was feeling defiant and wasn't a bit afraid of these guys. All they can do is arrest me, he thought.

Short cop stepped back a little, as if to give himself more room to move, and said, "If you don't leave now, I'm going to arrest you and charge you with criminal trespass." Matt just stood and looked at him, but said nothing.

Short cop gave the taller one a slight nod, which made the young officer spring into action. "You're under arrest for criminal trespass. Put your hands behind your back." Matt did as he was told. With the alacrity of someone who'd done this many times before, the tall cop expertly clamped handcuffs onto Matt's wrists.

He was hustled out of the lobby with Short Cop leading the way, and Tall Cop moving Matt along swiftly behind. As he passed the manager, he could hear him say, "I told you I was going to call the cops." Matt ignored him and allowed himself to be put into the squad car. He was thinking about who he would call to bail him out in the morning. He could call his parents, but they weren't on such good terms since he'd moved out—his mother, especially. She was pretty vocal about how she felt about his decision to leave. She was even more upset when Jesse came to help him move his stuff. That had been three months ago, and he'd barely spoken to them since. Even so, he figured enough time had passed for them to cool off, and they would be glad to see him, even under these circumstances. He'd have to eat a little crow, but they'd eventually help him out.

With those pleasant thoughts in his head, Matt leaned back in the squad car and closed his eyes. Now that he had a plan, he was able to relax a little. He realized now how tired he was and looked forward to getting booked so he could get some sleep in his cell. Everything will be alright in the morning, he thought as he drifted off…

CHAPTER 12

The Fight

J esse Carter was infuriated. He had just witnessed his friend Matt selling the Gypsy Gibson CD's he'd spent money to make, to patrons before their show at Peabody's, and pocketing the money.

For the past two years, he and Matt had worked hard to bring Matt's dream of forming a band into fruition. Matt had written the music and lyrics to a number of songs, and he'd come to Jesse to help him record his music. Jesse felt he was the "tech expert" between the two of them, and he knew Matt would need his knowledge to record his songs. "The Gypsy Gibsons wouldn't even exist without me," he thought, and he was probably right.

The two had played in a high school talent show together

and knew of each other's talents, so when Matt approached Jesse about collaborating, it seemed like a natural progression. Jesse had slaved over the process of recording the songs on those CD's; Matt was obsessed with getting each song exactly right, which made for exhausting sessions. "Matt would want to go over each song with a fine-toothed comb. Sometimes, we'd spend hours on one song. He knew how he heard it in his head, and until it sounded that way, at least to him, we'd have to keep going," Jesse later said.

He had put as much work into producing the music as Matt did making it, not to mention the money he'd spent. 'How dare he try to cut me out of my share! The nerve of that guy!' He was fuming. Didn't he let Matt move in with him when he wanted to leave home? He had even withstood the wrath of his mother as she cussed at him for helping her son move out.

Jesse got more and more angry as he played out in his mind the different times Matt had taken advantage of his generosity.

A few weeks prior to this show, the Gypsy Gibsons were scheduled to play the Odeon in the Flats, a popular club on the east bank of the Cuyahoga River in downtown Cleveland. Because they were a new band, promotion of their show would be left to them. Matt had assured the club manager they would be able to handle that. However, when told they had to pay for the tickets upfront, and then sell them to their fans for profit, Matt turned to Jesse for the funds.

"I shelled out the money for $500 worth of tickets. Matt, as always, was very persuasive, and I thought I'd make my money back," Jesse told me later. They couldn't sell anywhere near the $500, so Jesse figured since he and Matt were roommates, and they got into this together, Matt would at least give him half of what was lost. But Matt never mentioned it, as if it never happened.

To make matters worse, this very morning he had put a $252 charge on his credit card to bail Matt out of jail so he could play in the show. His parents were still pissed at him for moving and wouldn't put up the funds, so Jesse did it. Matt was the face of the Gypsy Gibsons, and his presence was integral. Once again he felt used by Matt as he watched him sell another CD and keep the money.

I'm going to get my money, or there's gonna be trouble for Matt Green, he thought. He was determined to get paid, and was going to confront Matt about it right now! Jesse didn't care about the show anymore; all he was focused on was making Matt pay up. He was so angry he hadn't noticed his fist clinched so tightly, the fingernails on each hand were almost cutting into his palms.

The other band members, Joe Revay, and Eric Harms, were setting up their equipment and doing sound checks, making sure their guitars and amps were on the right settings. Matt was busy chatting up the guests when Jesse approached with a pugnacious look in his eyes. "Matt you owe me money, and I want it NOW! I saw you selling those CD's and put the money in your pocket. I want my fuckin' money right now!" he yelled at Matt.

Matt seemed unphased by Jesse's obvious anger. He looked at him and said, almost nonchalantly, "If it wasn't for my music those CDs would be worthless. I have every right to sell them, and keep the money." That was the last straw, and without another word, Jesse lunged at Matt. This caught him a little off guard, but Matt managed to keep him at arm's length until the club security broke it up. The loud commotion must have alerted the bouncers, and they quickly escorted the combatants out of the building.

Matt's best friend, Sam Sizemore, freshly back from Spain after being gone two years, came to show support for his friends. "When I came back from Spain, Matt had the Gypsy Gibsons together, and I was impressed, if not a little envious. But I have to admit, I'd never seen a band get kicked out of their own sound check before," he would tell me later.

By this time, Jesse was absolutely livid! Once they were outside, their argument continued. "You're gonna pay me my money or else!", he spat the words at Matt.

"I'm not giving you anything. It's my music, and that means it's my money," Matt said, and started laughing with Joe and Eric. This incensed him even more, and he stormed off to his car.

Matt, Joe, Eric, Sam, and a friend of theirs, Jeff Peters, with his girlfriend, were all hanging out in Peabody's parking lot discussing what had just transpired. All of a sudden, Joe looked up and saw Jesse rounding the corner of the building, wildly swinging a baseball bat. "Heads up guys. Jesse's comin' with a bat!" he told the others, and you could visibly see Joe steeling himself, getting ready for battle.

As he got closer, they could see Jesse's eyes locked on Matt, bad intentions in his stare, continuing to swing the bat indiscriminately at anyone who got between him and his intended target. "I want my fuckin' money!" he yelled. One of his errant swings nearly hit Jeff's girlfriend, causing everyone to be in attack mode, but only this time, it was directed toward Jesse.

Eric struck first, hurling an almost full two-liter beer bottle in Jesse's direction. His aim was surprisingly accurate, hitting Jesse hard in the head with a resounding smack. Incredibly, this distraction didn't slow him down as he managed to get by Eric's two-liter assaults, and headed straight for Matt. Tears of fury were coming from his eyes, his mouth in a gaping rictus, flailing his bat as he got closer to his adversary.

Jeff's girlfriend, figuring he wouldn't intentionally harm a girl, tried to reason with him. "Jesse put the bat down. Please, you're not being rational." As if to let her know he would indeed "harm a girl," he swung the bat a few times at her, coming close to actually hitting her. She stepped back out of the way, and finally he saw a clear path to Matt.

Matt was watching Jesse coming at him with the bat, taking practice swings as if he were a major league batter on deck. He could hear the whooshing sound the bat made as it tore through the air, inches from his head. Joe, Eric, and Jeff stood around the two combatants ready to pounce, but couldn't get too close while he was swinging away.

Matt kept Jesse and his Louisville slugger at bay by circling him, but being careful not to get within the bats radius. He started gauging how much time between swings, and noticed Jesse was losing velocity after each one. "He's getting tired," Matt thought, and immediately devised a plan.

Jesse was so focused on hitting Matt with the bat, and up to now, watching him back away, that he was caught by surprise when Matt moved in close. "I've got him now," thought Jesse as he swung once more, aiming for a solid body blow. However, all the energy he'd expended up to now, blindly swinging but hitting nothing, had taken most of the steam off of his bat. By the time the bat reached Matt, he had nimbly moved to within a foot of Jesse, trapping the bat to his body with his left arm, the blow mostly ineffectual.

With a twist of his arm and a shove to Jesse's chest, Matt wrenched the bat from his hands and stepped back, ready to turn the tables on him with his own weapon. However, Matt never got the chance because as soon as Jesse was disarmed, Joe, Eric, and Jeff jumped into the fray, pummeling him to the ground. Shoes were coming off feet, as they started administering kicks to Jesse's legs and torso.

"I felt sorry for Jesse," said Sam. "He was crying, and I really felt bad for him. Luckily, a homeless guy broke the fight up or he would have really gotten hurt."

Exhausted and outnumbered, Jesse knew this was a battle he couldn't win. Still angry, but bruised, he decided it was in his best interest to get the hell out of there. He managed to get to his feet and make a hasty retreat to his car. "Fuck those guys, and fuck the Gypsy Gibsons!" he thought as he started his car to leave. He knew at that moment, he never wanted to see Matt ever again. He resolved to totally disassociate himself from the Gyspy Gibsons, and Matt specifically. Since Matt had moved in with him, he felt it was his right to evict him. He began to feel better with this knowledge. "I hope he saved some of that money he owes me, 'cause he's gonna need it to find another place to live," he chuckled to himself as he prepared for life without Matt and the Gypsy Gibsons.

Back at Peabody's parking lot, the band, minus Jesse, were discussing what had just happened. "None of us would have jumped in if he didn't have that bat," said Joe Revay. Meanwhile, Eric looked at Matt, who was still holding the bat, and said, "Gimme that bat." Once it was handed over, Eric gave a mighty heave, and threw the bat onto Peabody's roof.

Joe would talk about it later to me, saying, "The way Jesse was being indiscriminate about who he was swinging at, even a girl, really got all our blood boiling."

What none of them knew at the time was Matt had not been taking his medication lately, believing the lethargic side effects would take away his musical edge. Since he'd left his parent's house, he knew he was free to do whatever he wanted. Even though he was aware of the consequences, he decided not to take any more medicine.

However, in doing so, he effectively ended his dream of being the leader of his own band. The Gypsy Gibsons short run was over, and without his medicine, he would continue spiraling into manic episodes.

Two months after the fight, Matt would once again be in jail.

CHAPTER 13

The Reception

*"I have to make sense of this chaotic plethora of intangible
miscellany I call, my mind."*

-Matt Green; written on a napkin in a Shaker Hts. jail-

It was a typical June summer day. The temperature was
in the 80's, and you could see waves of heat rising up
from the asphalt on the streets. On such a sultry day, residents
of the Coventry area of Cleveland Heights were leisurely
window shopping at the many stores that lined both sides
of Coventry Road, the social center of the city. An eclectic
array of clothing stores, coffee shops, restaurants and bars
are located within a few blocks of each other. The pedestrians
milling about the sidewalks are as diverse as the storefronts
they pass. All ethnic types can be seen as one sits at the many
seating areas situated in front of eating establishments and
bars.

Doug Dixon was one of those people seated there, having a cold beer and watching the many pretty young ladies passing in front of him. Blonds, brunettes, short, tall, and the exotic, were all out, enjoying the cooler temperatures of the early evening. An added bonus for Doug was that the heat from earlier in the day had the ladies wearing clothing that covered only what was necessary to not be considered obscene. Ah, thank God for hot weather, he thought.

While admiring the posterior of a particularly well-endowed blond, he happened to notice a tall, wild-eyed young man lurching toward his table. Doug watched him a little more closely to see what he was up to. It appeared the guy was confused, and apprehensive. He also noticed every time someone would walk too close to him, he'd recoil suddenly, as if he were expecting that person to take a swing at him. His eyes were wide and constantly moving from side to side, as if perpetually searching for that elusive adversary.

As the guy got closer, Dave thought he looked familiar. He looked like a guy named Matt he'd seen before but couldn't remember where. He decided to help him because he was obviously distressed in some way. He could see the guy was paranoid and probably high on something. The dude had stopped walking, and stood with his back against the wall of a building about ten feet away, his head moving around as if on a swivel.

Dave finished his beer, gathered himself, and approached

the person he knew only as Matt. As he got closer, he could see the young man was quietly talking to himself, his eyes still surveying all who got close to him.

"Hey man, are you alright?" he asked. The guy didn't say anything, but eyed him suspiciously. He tried another tactic. "Is your name Matt?"

This seemed to bring the young man out of his stupor, and he said, "Yes, I'm Matt.".

'Good,' Dave thought. 'I'm getting through.' "Dude, are you feeling alright?" he asked again.

Matt looked at him for a long moment then said, "I'm trippin', but I'm alright."

Now Doug knew where he'd met Matt before. He'd seen him with Dave Hancock, an acquaintance of his, notorious for getting high all the time. If Matt was anything like Hancock, he was definitely high on something… and it wasn't just weed.

"Okay that's cool, but do you have someone you can call to pick you up, 'cause if you're trippin' as hard as I think you are, someone may notice and call the cops," Doug told him.

Matt took out his phone and said, "I'm gonna call my friend Malcolm Regan." Doug, coincidentally, knew Malcolm well, and asked Matt to hand him the phone so he could talk to him.

Once Matt had made the connection, he gave him the phone. "Hey Malcolm, it's Doug. I'm here with Matt, and he's high on something and acting really weird. Can you come pick him up? I don't want someone to call the cops."

Malcolm said, "I can't right now. I'm at a wedding reception at my ex's house in Shaker Heights. Plus, I don't have enough gas to get over there. Can you bring him here?"

Doug agreed to bring Matt to the reception but had his reservations. He wasn't sure if that was such a good idea, considering Matt's state of mind. However, Malcolm seemed to be comfortable with it, so why should he worry. All he'd do is take him there and be on his way. How hard could that be?

Little did Doug know at the time, Malcolm was thinking about that too. He and Matt had been good friends for a long time. He'd seen him high, and "acting weird" many times before, but he was always harmless. Nothing ever happened that caused anyone alarm when he was "that way." What could go wrong?

On the way to the reception, Dixon was able to get some lucidity from Matt. During those moments, Matt told an interesting story about how he came to be in this situation.

Apparently, he'd been at a friend named Naomi's house. Her parents weren't home, so she invited Matt to come over to "get high on acid." "We were having a great time, drinking and tripping off the acid, when her mother came home unexpectedly," he said. Being caught with a boy in the house while she was away caused Naomi's mom to go "ballistic"!

According to Matt, a lot of yelling ensued between Naomi and her mother, and in the confusion, he was able to make it out of the house and onto the streets. Hallucinating on the acid, and paranoid to the extreme, he finally made his way to Coventry, where Doug saw him.

After telling his story, Matt fell silent for the rest of the ride. When they drove up to the house, about fifteen minutes later, Doug could see Matt become agitated, looking all around as if he were expecting someone, or something, to jump out at him. "Where are we?" he asked. Doug told him they were about to hook up with Malcolm, which seemed to relax him enough to get him out of the car.

When Doug saw Malcolm, he hustled Matt over, gave him the details of what Matt had told him, said "Good Luck," and was out of there faster than a greyhound at the dog races.

Malcolm looked at his friend Matt for a long time. He was somewhat unsettled by what he saw. Here was this person who usually had it all together; great musician, incredibly intelligent, and able to adapt socially to any situation. Now, he was obviously high on some serious drugs, suspicious of everyone, and making erratic movements as he stood observing the people gathered in the room.

The reception was in full swing. There was a string quartet supplying soft music, food was in abundance, and the drinks were flowing. The fifty or so guests were enjoying the relaxed atmosphere, and chatting amiably among themselves.

Malcolm took Matt to the bar, thinking it would make him less tense if he had a drink. On the contrary, it only seemed to make him even more paranoid.

"He started doing really weird things. He became defensive and didn't want anybody near him, or touching him," Malcolm recalled. "Actually, I thought all the stuff he was doing was totally awesome! I really didn't want to be there anyway, so it was a great distraction." He thought Matt making all those straight-laced people nervous, was "incredibly cool."

After about an hour of "emitting strange energy" into the room, Matt suddenly got up from where he was sitting. According to Malcolm, he grabbed an empty bottle from one of the tables, whipped out his "green mile," and started pissing in it. "Right in the middle of the room!" said Malcolm. The guests were appalled, to say the least. Naturally, the parents of the bride, whose house it was, wanted him gone immediately; the young male guests were ready to take action and kick some Matt Green ass! A young lady there who happened to know him, and whom Matt, coincidentally, had a major crush on, offered to take Matt outside for a walk to calm him, and the situation, down.

Still tripping on the acid, and possibly in the throes of a manic episode, he refused to go with her, or anybody else for that matter. No one was going to take him anywhere, and he let it be unequivocally known. He'd previously told Malcolm he thought people were trying to kill him. The reason he'd used the bottle was because when he went into the bathroom, he thought snipers were outside the window, and he didn't want to get shot.

By this time, the male guests had seen enough, and decided to take matters into their own hands. They posse'd up, bum-rushing Matt, overpowering him, and carrying him struggling outside. They had every intention of giving him a solid thrashing. Rain had started to fall, covering the grass, and the antagonists, with a slippery sheen of moisture. This made it difficult to hold onto someone who had the advantage of possessing chemically induced strength.

Within a few seconds of being brought outside, Matt managed to wriggle free of his captors and ran off through the backyards of the neighboring houses. "Matt took off running with those guys chasing him through the yards. They were slipping and falling trying to keep up, but they eventually lost him," said Malcolm. During the commotion, someone had called the Shaker Heights police, and they were on the scene within minutes of Matt making his escape.

By this time, Malcolm was getting the "stink-eye" from the family and guests. "The family didn't like me anyway, and now I brought this dude who was causing all this trouble. It was a bad scene, but I really enjoyed it!" he said. The police were given the general direction of Matt's exit and went off to apprehend him. They eventually caught him on a nearby street. Because of his altered state of mind, he thought they were there to kill him, so he put up a fight with the cops.

This turned out to be his undoing. During the struggle, and while they were attempting to handcuff him, he somehow got his knee dislocated. This didn't deter him from trying to kick out the back window of the police cruiser, once they had him in the car. They returned to the reception to get statements from the homeowners, and took Matt to nearby Southe Pointe Hospital to get emergency treatment for his injury.

I was awakened from a sound sleep by the ringing of the phone. I looked at the clock, and the glowing numbers on the bedside digital clock said it was 1:30 am. Still half asleep, I answer with a gravelly "hello."

"Mr. Green?" a stentorian voice said. After confirming I was indeed Mr. Green, the voice continued. "This is the Shaker Heights police. Your son Matthew has been arrested for disorderly conduct while intoxicated, and resisting arrest. He's presently at Southe Pointe Hospital because he sustained a knee injury while struggling with our officers. If you'd care to come to the hospital to see him, now would be the time to do so. As soon as the doctor says he's okay to walk, at least with crutches, we're taking him to be booked at our station.

He said all of this in about twenty seconds, but it seemed much longer. I was stunned and couldn't think of anything to say, so I was silent. "Are you still there Mr. Green?" he asked. "Yes, yes, I'll be there. Thank you for calling," I said, thinking how wimpy I sounded.

What the hell have you done now Matt? I could see all his other "episodes" come crashing back into my consciousness, wondering what had triggered this one. Usually, it was because he hadn't taken his medication, but never had the police been involved before. This was different. I woke up Lynda and told her Matt was in trouble with the police and was at the hospital. "The hospital? What happened? Is he alright?" she was frantic.

"I don't know exactly. I just know he's at Southe Pointe, and we have to go, now!"

About a half hour later, we were led into the room where Matt was being held. His leg was elevated and his knee was heavily wrapped in what looked like ace bandages. He was also handcuffed to the rail of the bed he was lying in. He looked up at us as we came into the room and said, "Hey dad. It looks like I messed up."

"Yeah, I guess you did," I agreed. "What happened Matt?"

"Those damn police broke my knee, that's what happened!" he said indignantly. I could tell he was still high on something, although I didn't know what at the time. I told him to be quiet and not to say anything else. "I'm going to talk to the officer, I'll be right back."

I left him in the room with Lynda and went to have a conversation with the officer in the hall. "So what is he being charged with?" I asked him. He pulled out a small notepad, looked at it and said, "He's being charged with disorderly conduct while intoxicated, and resisting arrest. He fought with the arresting officers, and it took three of us to hold him down long enough to be handcuffed."

"Was he drunk?" I asked.

The officer had a little smirk when he said, "He admitted to drinking vodka and smoking marijuana, but the way he was struggling with us, I'd say he was on something a lot stronger."

He ended our conversation with, "We've been told by the attending physician he's been stabilized, so we can take him to the station. You and your wife should say your goodbyes to him now." I went back into the room and told Lynda the information I'd been given, all the while talking low, so Matt wouldn't hear me. Then, I went over to my son and said, "Listen, Matt. They're gonna take you to Shaker Hts. Police station to be booked, but I'll be there tomorrow to post bail. You're gonna have to come back home after this. No more of this foolishness, do you understand?" He looked at me sheepishly and nodded his head.

We kissed him, told him we loved him, and left the hospital. We had no idea this was only the beginning of his many forays into a life of extraordinary highs and lows, and his determination to do things his way, no matter the consequences!

CHAPTER 14

Crossroad

"Some guy called me on behalf of Verizon, to collect my debt. I told him that I was destitute, and disabled. He seemed to not hear me, because he continued on to give me payment options".

-Matt Green, notebook journal-

In the two years since the acrimonious fight with Jesse Carter, and the ensuing break-up of the Gypsy Gibsons, Matt was feeling anxious. When he left home to move in with Jesse, he had saved some money from a previous summer job and was five months away from graduation. Life is good, and the sky's the limit, he thought.

Then the bottom dropped out. Jesse indeed kicked him out of the Archer house. If it wasn't for his friend Kevin Warner, he would've had to show his parents he couldn't live on his own. Moving back in with them? Unacceptable. Kevin had been living out of his car, after being kicked out by his parents, and offered Matt his 'hospitality' for as long as he needed it. Matt and Kevin withstood the harshness of a cold Cleveland winter, before splitting up in the spring.

When reflecting on that time years later, Kevin would stare off into space, and with a little smile say, "That was one of the best times in my life. We didn't think it was so bad, and both of us really enjoyed our long talks in that car." Matt moved in with his friend, Dave Hancock, after he and Kevin mutually agreed to part ways. Kevin had found his own accommodations.

It was during this time that Matt started experimenting with different drugs to self-medicate. He felt the "beans" he had to take to control his mood swings had too many side-effects that took away his "edge." He'd decided when he left home, he would stop taking the medicine periodically, especially if he needed to concentrate. Besides, nobody knew exactly how he felt, even when he wasn't having an episode, so why listen to what anybody thought? His early introduction to philosophy during his punk years, and later, his exposure to Sartre, and Schopenhauer, had Matt well prepared to do things his own way... as an existentialist. "Man is a product of his own creation," I overheard him saying to someone while on the phone, "So if that's the case, I'm going to create my own reality. One where I decide what's best for me."

However, having made that decision, he never anticipated

the dangers of having that attitude during a manic episode. Add to that being high on something, and you had the perfect storm for law enforcement intervention. Which is what happened at the reception, and why he was back with his folks, which explained his anxious feeling.

He'd tried going to the local community college, and was doing quite well, if he had to say so himself. However, the stress of mid-term exams began to increase his anxiety level, and abracadabra, like magic, up pops Mr. Episode! Now he was kicked out of Tri-C, barred from returning for a year. He had no money, and no job prospects (he really didn't want to work for anyone other than himself, so he wasn't looking). He knew there had to be other ways to get money. He just didn't realize the solution to his problem was right in the house all the time, in the form of his grandmother.

"Grandma Green," had been living with them since his parents bought the house, and her sage wisdom comforted him most when he felt overwhelmed. One day, shortly after being released from his last hospitalization, Matt decided to talk to her. "Grandma, I'm 20 years old, and I'm no closer to being on my own than I was before I left home. I don't have any money, and no way to get any…at least legally, and I don't know what else to do. Mom and dad want me to get a job, but I can't work a steady job while I'm having these 'problems'."

His grandmother said, "Come here, Matt. You look like you can use a big hug!" He happily walked over to the recliner where she was seated, and dropped to his knees, allowing her to embrace him in the best hug ever! He would have gladly stayed in her arms for eternity.

All too quickly, the hug was over, and she sat back in her recliner. He stayed where he was, on his knees, so he could be at eye level when she talked to him.

"You know something, Matt? You've just answered your own question." She continued, "You may not be able to keep a job because of your 'problem', but because you have that problem will get you a check. What you have is a legitimate disability, and the gov'ment has to pay you for it."

Matt couldn't believe what he was hearing. Did she mean having bipolar disorder gave him the right to a check? "Come on Grandma, what's the catch?" he said. She smiled and said, "No catch, son. I'm gettin' a check because I have mental illness too. It's the law, boy."

He loved his grandmother, but she could sometimes get her facts mixed up. It's not that she was lying; she just believed what she said to be true. Whether it was or not didn't really matter to her. So naturally, he did his own research, and sure enough, she was absolutely correct! Under the Americans with Disabilities Act of 1990, there was indeed a law that allowed people diagnosed with certain mental illnesses to receive a Social Security Disability benefit, ergo, money! Right then, he decided to do whatever he needed to do to get that check!

Matt made up his mind not to take any more medication

until he went to the Social Security office. He felt he needed to be alert when he went to apply for assistance. After all, he was the one who had the most to lose if something went wrong. He wasn't going to let the meds be the reason for that happening. "I'm not going in there all 'zombied up', he thought.

For the next two weeks, Matt took his medication only once. He knew the dangers of not taking it daily, but he was convinced he could control his behavior. At least long enough to check on his benefit eligibility. Besides, he thought it would be to his advantage if he showed up somewhat "out of sorts." "If I'm applying for benefits, they need to see why," he reasoned. He just hoped he wouldn't have a relapse before he went to his appointment.

CHAPTER 15

Matt, S.S.I, & Mr. Gore

"Destitution, mental health issues – these are the makings of a genuine struggle. My struggle. It feels good to have a struggle."

-Matt Green-

PART 1

As we pulled into the parking lot of the local Social Security Administration building, Matt was slouched in the passenger, seat with his headphones on. His IPod was positioned in the console of the SUV, and I'd watched as he periodically picked it up to change the settings. He hadn't said anything during the ride, until we got out of the car. "I'm not going in." I was already headed toward the building when I heard his monotone voice.

I turned to ask him why, but the look on his face made me hesitate. His eyes were wide with … fear? His complexion was pale, and it looked as if he was slightly trembling. "Matt, what's the matter?"

"I'm not going in there. They're gonna lock me up," he had total conviction in his voice. Matt had been hospitalized twice in the past two months. When he was discharged the last time, I could tell he wasn't quite himself, but I attributed it to the side effects of his medication. Now, I knew he was either about to have an episode or was right in the middle of one. I walked back to where he was standing by the car.

"Listen Matt, all we're going to do is go in and talk to someone about getting you benefits. No one's going to lock you up, I swear." I could see he was mulling it over, but he still didn't move. I decided to use a ploy I'd tried before, when he was being episodically recalcitrant. "Okay, I'll tell you what I'll do. I'll go in first to check it out. I'll make sure I tell everyone not to lock you up. I'll be right there next to you all the time, to make sure they don't." I tried to sound as convincing as possible.

Normally, I'd get an earful from Matt about how absurd that sounded, how I must think he's a moron. But today, in his state of mind, my idea must have had merit. I could see him relax a little then he said, "Okay, go check it out."

I walked to the main entrance, looking back once to make sure he didn't run for it. He was still standing there, but I could see I'd better not take too long. He looked ready to bolt at any minute. I'll just go in long enough to look around, and make him think I'd fulfilled my mission.

Even though it was 8 a.m., the number of people waiting to be seen by a case worker let me know I wasn't the only one thinking "the early bird catches the worm." There must have been thirty or more crowded into the small reception area. A lone security guard was seated at a desk to the left of the entrance. He checked everyone's I.D. before allowing them to take a number from the ticket dispenser, located on the corner of his desk.

I took an extra few minutes before heading back out to where Matt was waiting. He didn't look frightened anymore, but he still had the air of apprehension about him. "Come on, Matt. I've let everyone know not to lock you up. I told them we were only here to get information, and then we'd be on our way," I said, trying to sound upbeat. He didn't say anything, just put his earphones back on and followed me into the building.

We found a spot in the back corner of the waiting area somewhat secluded from the rest of the people in the room. I could tell Matt's paranoia was kicking in because he kept looking around the room, as if expecting someone to come after him. He was tense as he sat in the chair, arms folded, his legs stretched out in front of him, crossed at the ankles. "Wait here while I go get a number for us," I told him, and walked over to the desk where the security guard watched me approach.

"I.D. please," he said. I gave it to him and told him I was

there on behalf of my son. "We're here to see if he qualifies for benefits," I said, pointing to Matt in the corner. The guard barely looked up as he handed back my I.D. and said, "Take a number and wait for it to be called." I thanked him and went back to sit with Matt. Once I sat down next to him, he seemed to totally relax, leaning his head back on the wall with his eyes closed.

While waiting, I thought back on the last several days... aggravating and tiresome, especially for Lynda. I'd noticed how he'd started antagonizing her, refusing to do anything she asked of him, stating he was too much of an "intellectual" to do menial chores. He'd also started correcting her when she mispronounced a word, or worse, mock the way she said it, laughing hysterically. "He's got to go back to the hospital, Rick. I don't think he's been taking his medication again." I was thinking the same thing. We could see he wasn't sleeping much, a sure sign he was on the verge of another relapse.

Indeed, he not only kept awake all day, but would walk the hallway between our bedrooms all night. He'd talk loudly on the phone, keeping Lynda and I from getting any sleep. His conversation was pressured, as if his mind was going 100 miles an hour, and he couldn't say the words he was thinking fast enough. His paranoia was heightened, and he would comment on how he thought we were out to get him. 'You're trying to take advantage of me, and I'm not going for it!" he told me once.

"What are you talking about, Matt?" I'd asked.

"You know exactly what I'm talking about!" he'd say, and run up to his room.

Just the night before, on one of the rare times we were able to sleep, Lynda told me she was awakened by an ominous feeling.

"When I woke up, my eyes took a while to get adjusted to the dark," she explained to me, "But when they did, I was startled to see Matt standing over me, on my side of the bed. I couldn't see his eyes, but I knew he was staring at me." Then, with a small shudder she said, "It was creepy because he wasn't moving, talking… nothing. Just standing there staring at me." She said she didn't want to wake me, so she quietly got out of bed, pushing him back as she did so. She then gently grabbed his arm, and pulled him out of the room. "He didn't resist or anything, he just let me take him back to his room, but I had to let him know I didn't like him coming into our room like that!" Secretly, Lynda was becoming afraid of her son.

Now here we were, with Matt in the midst of a bout with psychosis, and paranoid to boot. Even though Matt seemed quiet and relaxed right now, I knew when our number was called, he would be on the defensive once more, and would not cooperate. By now, I was very familiar with the signs and symptoms of his bipolar episodes. I felt sure this was the calm before the storm.

Finally, after about a forty-five-minute wait, our number was called. "Matt wake up." I shook his arm, not sure if he was dozing. "I'm not sleep. I just had my eyes closed," he said with a hint of anger in his tone. I was really concerned now and said, "Are you sure you're ready for this? We can come back another time, when you feel better."

He snatched the ticket from my hand, saying, "I can handle it. Just watch." His earlier fears about someone locking him up seemed to have disappeared, as he walked confidently to the window of the case worker who called our number. Maybe I was wrong, I thought, but I still went to the window with him to make sure things went without a hitch.

The case worker's name was Mr. Gore. He was a black man of average height, with a well-kept beard. He was a little overweight, with a pretty impressive beer belly protruding over his belt. He shook our hands and told us to follow him to his office. Calling where we went an "office," would be generous. It wasn't really an office at all, but a small cubicle. There was barely enough room for the small desk, and the two folding chairs positioned in front of it. "Sit down, please," Mr. Gore said, and started pulling out forms from one of the desk drawers. He handed one to Matt and said, "Fill out the highlighted areas, then we'll talk after you've finished"

I was watching Matt carefully, to see what his reaction would be, but he was watching Mr. Gore just as closely. The social worker wasn't aware he was being stared at as he was busy writing on one of the forms he'd taken from his desk. I noticed a bald spot at the top of his head, which I hadn't noticed before. He had a full Afro. Matt hadn't picked up the pen on the desk, or even attempted to fill out the form. He just kept staring at Mr. Gore.

Not sensing any movement from our side of the desk, he finally looked up to see Matt staring at him. "Is something wrong, Matthew? Do you need any help?" Matt didn't answer, he just kept staring at him.

I could see Mr. Gore was getting a little uneasy, so I turned to Matt and said, "Hey buddy, what's the matter?" Matt finally broke his stare on the social worker, and said to me, "Dad, would you mind leaving me and Mr. Gore alone? I don't need you to be here."

I was taken aback by this sudden change in his demeanor. "Are you sure, Matt?" I wasn't ready to leave him unaccompanied.

"I'm sure, dad. I'll be okay." Gore, unaware of Matt's condition, chimed in reassuringly. "It's okay, Mr. Green. I'll walk him through the application process to see if he qualifies for benefits. We won't be very long."

My better judgement told me to stay there with them. However, Matt had become very adept at covering up his psychosis for short periods of time—when he needed to. I sincerely hoped this was one of those times. "Alright. I'll wait outside," I said, and reluctantly left the cubicle for the waiting area.

PART 2

While watching Gore writing on a form on his desk, Matt instantly disliked the man. He wasn't quite sure why, but in his frame of mind, he just knew this guy was out to get him. On the verge of another manic episode, he decided he wouldn't cooperate with anything Gore wanted him to do... anything. He didn't want his dad to be here when he gave Mr. Gore the business, so he devised the plan to get him to leave. Matt knew because he was an adult, he didn't have to be hovered over by his parents anymore. At twenty years old, unless he was shown to be a threat to himself, or others, he was free to refuse medication, or have parent or guardian interference, if he chose.

So far, he was maintaining the appearance of keeping it together, although he suspected his father knew otherwise. He was feeling very agitated, and his thoughts were racing. He had trouble focusing on anything specific, but in his mind, he felt he was sharp as a tack.

The relentless pull of ensuing psychosis was overwhelming. However, he was comfortable in the now familiar sway of what he called, "that annoying exhilaration." He really didn't like when it was happening, but to him, it was an experience that had to be seen through. "This whole mental illness thing is a sort of experiment, and in the process, I'm figuring myself out," he wrote in one of his notebook journals.

Well, he was about to see where this particular "experiment" would lead. He was in a manic high and was ready to give this guy a hard time, something Matt truly believed Gore deserved. He looked over at Gore with a blank stare, and continued to do so, until Gore noticed no movement on the other side of his desk. He looked up.

"Well Matthew, is there anything you'd like to ask me?" Gore said, cheerily. Matt was silent a long time, and continued to stare at the social worker. Finally, after a good 30 seconds of silence, Matt said, "I don't see why I have to fill out anything. Isn't that your job?"

Gore was a little surprised by the question, but regrouped instantly. "Well Matthew, our policy is, if the applicant wants to get benefits, the applicant should fill out his, or her, own application." Gore laughed a little at his own joke, but cut it off when Matt didn't laugh with him. "So, if you don't mind, would you please fill out the form?" This guy was starting to give Gore the creeps.

Matt looked down at the papers, paused a moment, then picked up the pen on Gore's desk. "Alright, I'll fill it out," Matt said, and picked up the clipboard with the application attached.

Gore inwardly breathed a sigh of relief. Matthew Green was one weird dude, he thought. He'd seen his share of "strange" applicants in more than ten years of doing this job, but this guy was different. Where the other weirdos were obviously so, and some even funny, this guy Green was on another level! His weirdness was more intimidating than funny. The way his eyes kept moving when he stared at him made Gore think Matt was trying to hypnotize, or worse, mesmerize him!

Not to mention, the way he got his father to leave made him wary of his intentions. He had to admit, this young man had put a scare into him. He wasn't so sure being alone with him was such a good idea. Now, watching Matt fill out the forms, Gore figured he was in the clear. His previous apprehensions were gone. I guess he knew not to cause a problem if he wanted help, thought Gore. He smiled slightly at his obvious people skills.

At the same time Gore was mentally patting himself on the back, Matt was thinking how easy it was to placate so-called "professionals." Just say and do whatever they ask, or at least seem to, and you had them eating out of your hand. "What an idiot," he thought, as he dutifully filled in the highlighted areas. "If he only knew what I have in mind for him"

After he'd finished filling in all the spaces on the form, (except one), Matt handed the form back to Gore. He sat back in his chair and crossed his legs, waiting for what was about to come next.

Gore perused the form carefully, nodding his head in the affirmative as he went along. When he came to the bottom of the form, he saw it wasn't signed and dated. "Matthew you forgot to sign and date this at the bottom. Other than that, everything looks in order. If you'll just sign and date it, we can move on to the next step." Matt didn't take the forms or say anything. He just gave Gore that creepy stare again.

Gore could see this wasn't going to be easy, but he had supreme confidence in his ability to work with difficult clients. He took a sterner approach. "Matthew, if you don't sign the form, I can't even consider your application. If I don't have your signature, you don't have benefits, so please sign it."

Matt was really enjoying this! He delighted in watching this guy squirm under his time-tested stare. It worked like a charm. Especially when he was feeling so vital. He decided to throw Gore another curve ball. He uncrossed his legs, and leaned forward in his chair. With a perfectly straight face he said, "I don't like you, Mr. Gore."

Gore blinked his eyes several times and scooted his chair back, away from the desk. He had no idea what was about to happen. He wasn't about to get rushed by this guy, and be stuck behind the desk, defenseless. "Mr. Green, it's okay if you don't like me. I'm fine with that. You don't have a job like mine and expect all the applicants to like you. But if you really don't like me, just sign the form, and you can be on your way.

If you qualify, you get benefits. Whether you like me or not has no bearing on that." He softened his tone, "Please, just sign and date the form, and you and your father can go."

He reached out his hand holding the clipboard, expecting Matt to take it. Instead, Matt looked down at the clipboard, and back at Gore. He was really feeling his oats now, and was ready for a little mental sparring.

"I don't like you because you're fat, and you have a perfect beard," Matt said softly.

Gore started blinking rapidly again, unable to follow where this was going. "Wh..what?", was all he could stammer out. Matt didn't let up.

"And you know that bald spot you've tried not to draw attention to by growing an afro? Well, maybe it's because you think too much," then he paused before saying, "About the wrong things, like trying to get me to sign that form." He then laughed heartily.

Gore had had enough. Nothing in his job classification said he had to take crap from this pompous asshole! "I'm going to get your father, wait here." He hurried toward the waiting area. "Yeah, go get him," Matt said loudly, "But it won't do you any good."

PART 3

I was sitting in the waiting area, reading a past issue of Sports Illustrated someone had left on the seat when I heard someone calling my name. "Mr. Green, we have a problem." I looked up to see a flustered-looking Mr. Gore, walking swiftly toward me.

"What's wrong?" I asked, already knowing it was Matt.

Gore had a look of startled confusion on his face when he said, "Your son won't sign the application for benefits form. When I asked him to, he started insulting me. Now, I'm aware he needs the help, but he's an adult, and by law, I can't file if he doesn't sign and date the form. Do you think he'll do it for you?" he almost pleaded.

My mind was already thinking of alternatives to Mr. Gore's unsuccessful attempts to get Matt to comply. Unlike Gore, I knew what I would be up against when Matt was having a manic episode. In his frame of mind, he was the most intelligent man in the world. With his superior will alone, he felt he could control any, and all, situations. The only problem was, he wouldn't listen to any rational discussions, or even consider his thinking was flawed. All he knew was how he felt, and how he felt was all that mattered.

"Mr. Gore, Matt is having a psychotic episode right now. I knew he was acting strangely, but I thought he was well enough to handle this. He's probably paranoid and thinks if he signs, you'll have him locked up. If that's the case, even I can't make him sign." I could see the deflated look come over Gore, so I said, "I'll go with you and see what I can do."

"Oh thank you, Mr. Green", Gore said, and turned to head back to his cubicle. I followed, thinking this could have been prevented if I had stayed with them. Oh well; no use crying over spilled milk. I'd just have to see for myself how far Matt had spiraled in this short time.

As we walked up to the cubicle, I could see Matt's long legs, crossed at the ankle, sticking out beyond the partition that served as a privacy wall. I came around it and saw Matt leaned back in his chair, eyes closed, headphones on, slowly snapping his fingers to the tune he was listening to.

"Matt, take off those headphones and pay attention." I shook him hard, and spoke loud enough for him to hear me. He sat up immediately and snatched his headphones off. "Tell me why you won't sign the form, Matt."

He looked disdainfully at Mr. Gore and said, "He wants to lock me up. If I sign that paper, he's going to have me locked up!" The look on his face as he glared at Gore had me a little worried, but I kept pushing.

"Listen, Matt. I told you I wouldn't let anyone lock you up, and I meant it. The only reason he wants you to sign is to start your application process. He can't do it if you don't sign." I picked up the clipboard and handed it to him. "Go ahead and sign it Matt, and then I'll take you home. No one's going to lock you up." He looked at me, then hatefully at

Gore, and finally, at the clipboard.

After a long pause, he took the clipboard from my hand. He sat it on the desk and said imperiously, "Give me a writing utensil, peasant!"

"Cut it out, Matt!" I was getting tired of his disrespectful attitude. "He's trying to help you. There's no need to be rude." Gore tentatively reached across the desk to hand Matt his pen. "Sign and date please," he said, "And I swear, you won't be locked up."

Matt took the pen and picked up the clipboard. He sat back in his chair as if he were going to sign the form. Suddenly, there was a change in his expression. A frown began to form on his face. When he looked up at me, there was that unmistakable look of anger in his eyes. "Both of you must think I'm stupid. I know you're in cahoots. You're trying to get me to sign myself into a lock up." The certainty in his voice let me know he actually believed it. I was about to say something, to try to persuade him that wasn't going to happen, when Gore cut in. "We are not locking you up Matthew."

Gore's voice was the catalyst for what happened next. "Liar!" Matt spat the word at him and threw the clipboard and pen in my direction, barely missing my head. Then, with unexpected quickness, he stood up and, using his arm, swept everything off Gore's desk onto the floor. Pens, pencils, papers, everything. Even a coffee mug with #1 Dad etched on the side was knocked to the floor, shattered.

Gore jumped out of his seat, fear and astonishment on his face. "This meeting is over!" he said. As he hurried from his desk, I could hear him say, "Either leave now, or I *will* have him locked up!" I was totally embarrassed, but I was also livid. Matt may have blown his only chance at getting financial and medical benefits. I had no idea how much weight they put on initial interviews, but I felt certain this incident was not going to go over well for Matt.

He stood next to me with a smug look on his face. "I told him I wasn't gonna sign it," he said arrogantly. I wanted to knock that look off his face right then, but I could see the front desk security guard headed our way, Mr. Gore following close behind. Chastising Matt would have to come later.

"Let's go, Matt. You've caused enough trouble." I grabbed him by the arm, and unceremoniously pulled him toward the main entrance. We were headed in the direction of the approaching security guard, and Gore. They must have seen the 'don't-fuck-with-me' look in my eyes because they both stepped back and let us pass. Matt still wasn't done with Gore, and as we hurried past, he said, "That's right. Step aside, peasant. Your king is coming through!" Gore just shook his head sadly, and turned away. The guard watched us closely, until we went out the door. All the while he kept his hand on the taser attached to his belt.

I couldn't contain my anger. Even though I knew Matt's behavior was a direct result of his bipolar disorder, a part of me blamed him for not taking his medication as he should. He knew better than anyone what would happen if he didn't, so why would he not do what was necessary to stay healthy? All the turmoil he'd taken Lynda and I through because of his illness, between hospitals and jail, or both, had come to a head.

"Get in the car, Matt." I was furious but tried to maintain my composure. After we'd driven about a mile from the place, I turned to him and said, "Well Matt, I hope you're happy. You may have messed up any chance you had of getting the benefits you need. I'm done trying to help you when you continue to not help yourself."

He just slouched further down in the passenger seat, put those damned headphones on again, and closed his eyes. He was purposely ignoring me, and this made me even angrier. I slammed on the brakes, causing Matt to jerk forward so hard, if he hadn't had his seatbelt on, he would have gone through the windshield.

I reached over and grabbed him by his coat collar, pulling his face close to mine. I wanted him to see my rage. "Matt, I've had it with your pompous attitude and rude behavior. Right now, I hate your ass!" He pulls away from my grip and sits back in his seat. Then, without looking my way he says, "Yeah, well I think you drink too much, and read too many horror stories." He then put his headphones back on.

I was exasperated, my anger gone. I was ashamed of

myself for losing my temper, and worried that Matt wouldn't get the help he so desperately needed. I saw the frightened look on Mr. Gore's face when Matt cleared his desk. I wasn't so sure he'd be willing to deal with us again, if ever.

I decided I'd wait a few days and call him back. I'd really have to make sure I profusely apologized to him on Matt's behalf, and hope he understood my dilemma. Meanwhile, I was going to let Matt's own actions determine his immediate future. If his past history was any indication, it wouldn't be very long before we'd see what that future would be.

Two weeks later, I was again in the office of Mr. Gore. I'd had the presence of mind to keep the form Matt had thrown, and gotten him to sign and date it, after he'd taken enough of his medication to be less paranoid. "I'm truly sorry for my son's actions, Mr. Gore. What you witnessed was why we were here in the first place. Please don't take what happened personal. He has bipolar disorder and without Social Security benefits, I'm afraid his well-being will be irreparably compromised."

I waited to hear his rejection, but it didn't come. Instead he said, "Mr. Green, you need all the help you can get. I'll try to expedite his claim, and hopefully, Matthew will get his first benefit check in the next couple of months. I know it must be difficult for you and your wife, that's why I've decided to help you."

Gore was as good as his word. Matt indeed got his first check within two months, and his medical card came a few days later. All of this couldn't have happened at a better time because the day he got his first check, he was admitted into St. Vincent Charity Hospital's psychiatric ward.

CHAPTER 16

Matt and Tom

"One should note that the entire reason, or purpose of Sam's and my 'bad blood' was the introduction of Tom Nicholson to the equation of our lives."

-Matt Green, 2007-

The fact that Matt was being admitted into St. Vincent Charity Hospital was no surprise considering the things he'd done in the months leading up to it. Matt was now firmly of the mind that self-medication was the answer to his bipolar episodes, and he was on a mission to find out which drug worked best. He was never a big drinker after his punk years, but now he was drinking constantly... and would write about it. For instance, take this line from one of his 2007 notebooks dated July of that year:

"Ran into Roselyn. She fed me liquor. This was a good thing. She also told us of parties and friends, and being kicked out of Kent. I personally don't mind that she was kicked out of Kent. I'm drunk. So much for objectivity." This was a week after being released from Marymount Hospital Psychiatric Ward.

He was an avid reader of existential philosophy, especially where man "being a product of his own making" was concerned. He'd decided long ago to live his life as close to this ideal as possible, considering the restrictions he felt he was under. He wasn't about to compromise his creativity to his music by taking pills he just knew would affect his musicianship. Not to mention, he was now unquestionably an adult, which meant unless he was a threat to himself, or others, no one could make him take meds, or force him to comply with anything his parents told him to do. "I could go live with one of my friends if I want," he'd tell them if they tried to push him to take his meds.

He'd never stopped smoking weed, but with his increase in drinking came an increase in cigarette smoking too. He was always "destitute," as he put it, so he couldn't buy the cigarettes he'd developed such a taste for. However, this didn't mean he couldn't smoke. On the contrary, he was usually around friends who did smoke, and he wasn't ashamed to bum as many as he could during their gatherings.

"He'd bum cigarettes so much we started calling him Squareman," said his friend, Jim Carol, "because he'd always say, 'Let me get a square, man'. You'd get so mad at him sometimes, but then he'd come around and act like nothing ever happened, and you couldn't stay mad anymore."

Matt had tried just about every popular drug there was. His sojourn into the punk scene five years earlier had taken his controlled substance virginity, so he already had an idea of what he was looking for. "When I became a teenager, I was introduced to drugs," he wrote, "primarily, marijuana. The euphoric high was very pleasant, but I desired something more than a harmless, giggling, high… I wanted to *hallucinate*." (Italics are mine).

He turned to LSD for a while, and really enjoyed it. "It was all I expected of the drug. I saw the world with brand new eyes, experiencing life, as a whole, as if I was just born." However, Matt wanted more from his friends, and the drugs he used. As mentioned earlier, Matt knew about drugs for many years before he turned twenty. In fact, he was introduced to heroin back then by an older girl, "Lilly," who was very much into it. He hadn't forgotten how it seemed to abate his mood swings, even during an episode, so he knew this was something he'd have to try again.

His friends knew of this and tried several times to talk him out of it. "We were all mad at Matt when we found out he was using heroin," said Colleen Allison, Sam's girlfriend, and Matt's closest female friend, "but he didn't seem to care." Matt was not going to be told when, or with what, to get high. The way he saw it, they didn't know what he was going through, or how to stop it, so who were they to dictate what was best for him?

Enter Tom Nicholson. He was a handsome young man with unkempt, thick dark hair he wore just below his collar. He was about 5 foot nine, with a bounce in his stride that made him seem taller. He was full of energy and had no limits; Matt's Caucasian double.

Tom was a casual friend to Sam, and he also played music. They'd run in the same circles before, but when Sam moved to Spain, he started getting in touch with Tom a little more on the internet. By the time Sam returned in 2005, he and Tom got together more frequently. Late that year, Sam introduced Matt to Tom. "I remember they both had such big egos," Tom would say later, "They were trying to compete to see who would make music with me, and they started getting on each other's nerves, but I could tell they were very good friends."

According to Sam, Matt gravitated to Tom almost immediately. "I brought him (Tom) over there because we were all gonna play music, and what ended up happening was, he and Tom became really close friends. That's when I stopped hanging around as much, because those two got on like flies on shit." What Sam didn't know at the time was Matt and Tom had more than music in common. "I knew he had mental illness, and I knew I had mental illness," Tom said later, "We both had mental illness. The only difference was, he recognized his before I recognized mine."

Matt had found his partner in crime, so to speak. Someone he could play music with, and talk about philosophy with, and most importantly, someone who understood what it was like to have bipolar episodes. He was also someone naive to the things Matt had experienced, and was eager to share in the adventures Matt described.

"This guy was into some interesting things, and the more I heard him talk, the more I became fascinated with the person that was Matt. He was so different, and interesting, more so than anybody I'd ever met. I just really wanted to get to know him," said Tom. "Besides, here was this black kid who played rock and roll. Usually, it's white kids doing that. This was crazy!"

Tom and Matt spent a lot of time together playing music and getting high, both of them reveling in each other's company. In Matt's case, he had someone who was a kindred spirit, and who was willing to let him control the direction of their relationship. Tom had found someone he looked up to, someone who "seemed to have so much more knowledge than anyone else around him."

Matt wrote about their unique connection. "Tom and I are almost one and the same kind of mind: over-read suburban intellectuals who are light years ahead of our 'peers.' What's more, if there was any sort of decadence that Tom couldn't throw himself into, head first, then I could find it for him.... and oh, I did."

By now, Matt had perfected a man-of-mystery persona and enjoyed watching others being uncomfortable with his not so politically correct conversation. Tom was intrigued by the way people hung onto every word, even when they didn't like what he said, as Matt talked about "all this heavy stuff" in social gatherings. As Tom would put it later, "To be honest, I had the same reaction that most people had of Matt... except to me, it was a good feeling. It was a feeling of intimidation. Not in a physical way, but intellectually. He always seemed to be the genius in the room." Tom was totally under Matt's influence.

One day, a few months prior to his admittance to St. Vincent Charity, Matt and Tom were driving around looking to have some fun. They'd smoked some marijuana and had a few beers, when out of nowhere, Matt said, "You know, Kurt Cobain used to do heroin." Tom was taken by surprise by the statement, but he knew Matt well enough to know he wouldn't bring something like heroin up, unless he had it on his mind already. He didn't know if Matt was testing him; indeed, he wasn't even sure if he was joking, but he continued the conversation.

"I've never done heroin before, Matt. Have you?"

"Of course. It's a cool experience," Matt replied nonchalantly, as if it were the most natural thing in the world.

Tom was intrigued by the subject and curious as well. This would be a good time to show Matt he could be just as sophisticated, so he asked the question he would later come to regret. "Do you know where to get some?" Matt knew he could get Tom to latch onto the idea of trying heroin. He, himself, was doing it off and on with "Lilly" for the past couple of years. Better than meds, he felt heroin quelled the demons that possessed him during his episodes. However, he didn't want to seem too anxious. He had to reel Tom in slowly. "I know where to get some, but I won't do it. I don't want you having any more bad habits," Matt said jokingly.

Tom wouldn't take no for an answer. "Come on, Matt. You can't tell me how cool it is without letting me see for myself." Matt shook his head.

"Forget it, Tom. I'm not doing it." Tom was starting to get annoyed. "You're always saying how life should be experienced, and that's what I'm trying to do now. You and I both know I can handle it. Besides, I've got some money."

That sparked Matt's interest. The real reason he'd said no to his friend was because he was broke. Money was something that always seemed to elude Matt. As shameless as he was about bumming cigarettes, he was even more so when letting his friends use their money for his pleasure. Since Tom had the money and was eager to try, Matt decided to relent. "Alright dude. I'll make a call, but I'm gonna make sure you don't do too much. I don't want you having a bad experience your first time trying it."

A phone call and a twenty-minute drive later, they pulled

into the driveway of Matt's friend, Lilly. Tom would describe Lilly as a "pretty blond chick with a smokin' hot stripper body." Matt knew she would have what they wanted, and he didn't waste much time on formalities. "Hey Lilly, I have someone here who'd like to try some H., and he has some money. What do you think?" Lilly, who was just about to indulge herself, was happy to have these guys here to get high with. Plus, the fact she could make some money made it even better.

For his part, Matt had his own ideas about why he wanted Tom to be with him when he "popped his hard drug cherry." Matt considered himself an "authority" on getting high and felt it was his duty to make sure his friend was broken in under his watchful eye. "I figured if he only hung out with me when he did it, then he wouldn't be taken under into addiction. I would monitor his use," he explained in one of his journals. "Well, that fell through when I almost died right in front of him."

"That night was probably the craziest night of my life," Tom would say later. "She went in a room and came out with heroin, acid, coke, and beer... all at once. Matt convinced me to do it all with them, and I did. We'd just finished doing all those drugs when Matt fell out."

From that previously mentioned journal, here is Matt's rendition of what happened:

"We had about a gram of heroin between us. I didn't keep up with how much I had taken, and overdosed in the middle of the night, for about 20 minutes. When I came to, I was still too high to fathom the seriousness of the matter. Neither Tom nor Lilly could stop saying, "Dude, are you alright? I kept thinking, and saying, yes, I'm alright. I didn't feel dope-sick achy, I wasn't puking, and my head felt nice. As far as I was concerned, I was fine."

Matt's plan to protect Tom from addiction failed miserably. After he'd passed out at Lilly's house, he wanted to show his friend he could handle it better their next time trying. They did heroin "about three or four times" together, but Matt soon tired of the nodding-out high the drug induced. According to Tom, "he never did it anymore with me, but after I'd been introduced to heroin, I was off and running!"

Matt and Tom would continue their close association over the summer of 2007, getting high, playing music, and, as Tom would put it, "We would get high and go look for chicks." Matt had a girl he'd had sex with before, whom Tom thought was attractive. "I told Matt I'd like to get with her too. So Matt set it up," said Tom, and according to him, "Since he'd done that for me, I introduced him to this woman I'd been messing with who was older."

Her name was "Crystal." She was almost twenty years older than both of them, and she was into being dominated. When they came to her house, Tom pulled her to the side and said, "Go over there and have sex with Matt." She sidled over to him and said in a sultry voice, "Tom has commanded me to have sex with you." Matt and Crystal went to her bedroom and enjoyed each other for about an hour. When they returned, Matt was exhausted, but satisfied.

He'd later tell me that was the scariest sex he'd ever had. When I asked him what was so scary about it, he said, "She wanted me to slap her, and pull her hair. She had me call her all kinds of names while we were having sex. But dad, that was a little too intense for me. I don't want to beat up a girl in order to have sex with her."

That didn't stop him from going back several more times to "beat up" Crystal. "After her and Matt got together, she didn't want anything to do with me, ever again," Tom said. However, after a month of uninhibited sex with this older woman, Matt decided to stop the relationship. "I couldn't keep up with her. She was draining my energy," he'd say to me later.

This didn't mean Matt was jaded by sex with Crystal. On the contrary, he now had more experience and was anxious to show his younger girlfriends something new. Matt was also on the verge of another manic episode, and was now using sex as his means of coping.

CHAPTER 17

Sexapades

"He (Tom) was responsible for my first sexcapade with a 37-year-old nymph. But I had a lot of fun before that!"

-Matt Green-

M att sat in the admitting area of St. Vincent Charity Hospital's Psychiatric ward, lustfully eyeing the pretty young nurse who'd just walked by. His parents had probated him because he'd been noncompliant with his medication for a few months. His erratic, often frightening behavior caused them to take drastic measures and get help from the court. They figured if he wouldn't listen to them, he'd have to comply with a court order.

The Bedford police, who'd had their share of trouble with Matt, willingly came to the house to arrest him. They unceremoniously handcuffed him and forcefully took him to the hospital. He knew he'd probably have to spend at least four days there. If that was the case, he'd have to figure out a way to have some fun while staying as a "guest." This was his third different facility, so he had a good idea of how things worked. 'Once you've seen one psyche ward, you've seen 'em all', he thought with a smile. This one was even better than the others for one reason. He could see there were at least two, maybe three, cute patients who were giving him the once-over.

In his manic state, Matt could only think about one thing… sex. He and Tom had spent the last month having uninhibited sexual encounters with an older woman, and he'd gotten used to the frequency of those events. However, once the "annoying exhilaration" took control, he was on automatic pilot. He zeroed in on one young patient in particular.

This is what Matt wrote about her:

"She had blond hair, almost white, that hung down to her shoulder blades. It looked so fair, when the light hit it the right way, you almost thought it was a halo. She had small, naturally red lips, the nemesis of lipstick. Those same lips smiled easily, and were almost heart-shaped. Her eyes defied her warm smile, as they were a cold blue. So light in color, they seemed to look right into your soul. Frightening, but intriguing."

He noticed when she stood up to walk, she maintained eye contact as she sauntered slowly to her room. Matt thought she was just his type, slim, but well put together. Tall, but not too much, with small, perky breasts that were braless under her flimsy shirt. Her hips moved fluidly, hypnotizing Matt, who was watching her intently.

'I think I just found my fun,,' was his first thought, but then he realized he was in a facility that watched you constantly, and closely. If he was going to get with the "ice queen," as he came to think of her, he'd have to be resourceful, and quick. He only had four days to accomplish his mission. He enjoyed the challenge, but in his state of mind, he knew he couldn't do what was necessary to make it happen.

His experience at the other facilities gave him some idea of how he might be able to pull it off. He already knew it would take at least two days for the initial combination of meds they gave him to work. That would stabilize his mood swings so he could trust himself enough to make conversation with her. Matt had told his brother Eddie, "my pimp hand is strong because my conversation is so compelling. I know I can get any girl to talk to me. Once they do, I've got 'em."

He felt the effect of the drugs pulling him into a pre-slumber haze, and welcomed it. He hadn't had more than an hour or two of good sleep in weeks, and he knew his body was about to shut down. Falling into a drug-induced sleep was just what the doctor ordered, literally, and he wasn't going to make a fuss about it. He would need his sleep if he was going to represent himself well before the "queen." He ambled to his assigned room (which was next door to his girl, by the way), and fell heavily into the well-worn mattress on the small bed. They'd given him a standard issue bathrobe and pajamas, which was to be worn day and night during his stay, so getting ready for bed was one action he didn't have to deal with. He was ready to sleep... long, and hard.

As he floated into the inevitable, his mind still on her, he reminisced about his first time, and the look on his dad's face, when he found out.

"Hey dad, girls are great!" That statement came when Matt was thirteen years old and already starting to be noticed around the neighborhood as the bad-boy skater/guitarist among the Bedford kids. He'd been hanging around the skaters since he'd moved to the city, but they were mostly boys his age. However, a year of intense daily practice on his guitar had made him good enough to play in front of friends. Some of the girls who hung with their crowd were apparently beginning to show an interest.

As an adolescent, Matt frequently talked to Sam about how undesirable he perceived himself to be. As if his eye problem wasn't enough, he'd developed a prominent overbite when his permanent teeth grew in. "He thought he was ugly, for sure, when he was younger," Sam remembered. This would cause him a lot of anxiety since he thought it might one day affect his love life.

"No girl would want to talk to someone with shifty eyes

and bucked teeth, dad. My life's so messed up." My heart broke for him, but I couldn't allow him to start down that potentially depressing road. All I could think to do was reiterate the positive things in his young life.

"You have so much going for you right now, son. You have excellent grades in school. Your teachers all tell us what a good student you are. You're turning into a pretty decent guitar player too. Your mother and I have noticed how much improvement you've made in a relatively short time. To get that good requires dedication and focus. How many kids your age can say they practice longer, and more consistently than you? None, I guarantee it. I don't think any one of your friends spend the kind of time you do practicing, and it shows. Most importantly, you have a family that loves you and supports you one hundred percent."

"So don't worry about the girls Matt. Once you've mastered that guitar, and joined a band, the girls will come. It doesn't matter if you're ugly or handsome. It's a well-known fact; musicians get the girls. Look at Keith Richards!" He smiled a little at my joke, but I wasn't sure if it had made a difference, until I heard him practicing even more diligently on his guitar. Slowly, I noticed a phone call or two coming from young girls asking for Matt. He would grab the cordless from my hand and run up the stairs with it. Sometimes, he would tie up the phone for hours during one of those calls.

Now, here he was, grinning like a Cheshire cat, saying

how "great" girls were. Even though he was only thirteen, I knew he was well-informed about sex. His older brothers John, who was twenty-two at the time, and Eddie, nineteen, already had carnal knowledge. Matt had the perfect teachers to instruct him on the nuances of getting laid. Eddie, especially, felt it was his duty to show his little brother the finer points of navigating the female mind to get quicker sexual results.

Knowing this, I just came out with the obvious question. "So are you saying they're great because you've had sex?"

With a sly smile, he said cryptically, "Maybe," and once again, ran up to his room. Shortly thereafter, I could hear him playing his guitar, with a little more alacrity, I might add!

As it turns out, my assumption was correct. Matt had been seeing a friend of Sam's and Colleen's named Janine. "Matt lost his virginity to Janine," Sam told me years later. "They were together for two or three months, which at that age, seemed like a long time." Then, after a moment of reflection he continued, "You know, in our circle of friends, at that age having sex was commonplace. But now, I look at thirteen-year-old kids and think, Jesus Christ, what the hell were we thinking?"

Matt's "maybe" said volumes to me, and I made it a point to talk to him about condoms, and safe sex, that very day. I knew my son was very intelligent for his age and could talk about subjects so varied our adult friends would spend hours conversing with him at social gatherings. However, now that the "seal was broken,," so to speak, his intelligence would not be coming from the head on his shoulders. Janine had aroused his prurient curiosity, and he was determined to explore this new sensation more.

Over the ensuing years, as his guitar skills improved, Matt's confidence with the girls grew. His association with the skaters had pretty much ended, but he'd found another group of outcasts to hang with. The Punk scene not only allowed him to play with like-minded musicians, but also enjoy the company of older female "fans" who were more experienced in the art of lovemaking.

It was during this time Matt started referring to his penis as "the Green Mile." When he was about fifteen, he said to me one day, "Hey dad, Eddie told me the men in our family are well-endowed. I don't know about you or him, but I sure am!" He then proceeded to pull down his pants to prove his point. Somewhat startled, I said, "Hold it, Matt! I don't need to see it. I believe you. Pull your pants back up."

He complied but kept talking. "I measured it, and I'm almost eight inches long!" He couldn't control his enthusiasm. "I'm sure the girls won't care if I'm not cute once they see what I'm packin'!" As mentioned, Matt's confidence around girls increased with his improved instrumental skills, and his popularity in the punk scene. Young adolescent girls were no challenge when he was being approached by older girls in their late teens.

As his friend and former bandmate, Joe Revay would say to me later, "It didn't matter if it was Halle Berry. Matt would go right up to her and start a conversation. He was fearless around girls."

Two years after his introduction to sex, Matt had enough experience to try his hand at deflowering a virgin. The opportunity came when he met Sarah Solomon. Sarah, a cute, bespectacled blond also in the Bedford punk scene, had started spending time with Matt more during high school. Matt's friend and Gypsy Gibson bandmate, Eric Harms, was a good friend of Sarah's, and set them up for the first time. Eric's brother, Greg Slawinski explains it this way:

"Eric set Matt and Sarah up after Matt kept bugging him about wanting to get with her. He called her up, and they eventually had sex. After a while though, they stopped dealing with each other. I never figured out why, but it seemed like they really disliked each other." Then, after a moment he said, "You know what's funny? Matt took her virginity, and I lost mine to her."

According to Sarah, "Matt was my first time. We were so young, I really had nothing to compare it to. Neither of us knew what we were doing." When asked were they dating, she would only say, "We were a little more than friends."

As Colleen would say later, "Matt and Sarah had a very physical relationship… it was pretty intense." After their graduation from high school, they drifted apart, but the die had been cast for Matt. His early sexual conquests made him increasingly bolder in his interactions with the girls. His natural curiosity compelled him to try new approaches to penetrate (pun intended) the female psyche.

"The dude had balls, I have to say that," said Greg Slawinski. "I remember he had some chick he knew come over. As soon as she came on my porch, Matt told her, 'So, you want to blow me?' I thought she'd be upset, but she said 'okay,' and got right down to it.... in front of everybody! Can you believe it?"

Matt's reputation with the girls was becoming legendary among his friends. He'd grown into a totally different person from the gangly awkward teen he once was. By the time he reached his twentieth birthday, he was a tall, strapping young man with a full beard. He'd always had a slim build, but because he'd started working out, was now sporting a body that was lean and muscular. He also subscribed to GQ magazine, looking to change his style into something more unique, but trendy. As Colleen would remember, "I hadn't seen Matt in a while, but when I did, he was totally different than I remembered. He was this tall, bearded, good-looking man who was a snappy dresser. I was impressed."

Matt had no shame when it came to showing off his new body either. "He'd ask any girl, even if he just met them, if they'd like to see his six-pack. Sometimes, they'd say no, but a lot of times they'd say yes! That dude had no fear around the chicks!" said Greg.

Also, around this time, Matt had developed a trick to get girls that, to his friends, seemed unthinkable. He would actually pull out the Green Mile for female inspection.

Greg Slawinski:

"Me, Matt, and a girl from the neighborhood were in her car driving to Matt's house to smoke. This girl always had good smoke, so we spent a lot of time with her. This particular day, we were in the car in Matt's driveway smoking and just shootin' the shit. All of a sudden, Matt says to her, 'I think my penis is too small. What do you think?' I thought she was going to be mad, but she said 'Okay Matt, let me see.' Matt was in the backseat behind me, so I couldn't see him, but I did see her eyes get real wide, and she gasped a little and said, 'Oh my God, Matt! Oh my God!'"

"I turn around and Matt has his dick out. I wasn't that surprised because I'd been around when he'd done that before, but I was surprised at her reaction. She couldn't take her eyes off it. Then Matt says, 'Do you want to suck it?' and she says, "Sure!' and they go behind Matt's garage. After a while, I went to check on them because they were taking so long. When I go back there, Matt's sitting on a tree stump, and she was on her knees going down on him... deep throat! Later, he told me she was like a Hoover vacuum. She sucked up everything."

Matt had become the "rock star" he always imagined

himself to be…at least in Bedford. Sex, drugs, and rock and roll, literally, was now his way of life, and he had no regrets.

CHAPTER 18

The Ice Queen Cometh

Matt woke from a sound sleep with a start. The single window in his small room showed no light outside, so he knew it was at least late evening. He was still sluggish from the meds he'd taken, but more importantly, he was able to organize his thoughts without the influence of the manic episode he came in with. 'Good,' he thought; 'the meds worked!' He still felt he could sleep some more, but he wanted to check out his surroundings first.

He relieved himself and rinsed out his dry mouth with several drinks of water from the sink. All he had for clothes was the robe and pajamas he was issued, so he decided to make himself as presentable as possible and head to the patient's common area. As he left his room, he heard a female voice say, "Well, sleeping beauty finally woke up, and I didn't even have to kiss him."

Matt turned around and was surprised, and delighted, to see the "ice queen" standing in the doorway of her room next door. She was holding a soda can and lounging lazily against the door frame, wearing the same hospital-issued pajamas and robe as his.

Even though he was still a little foggy, he felt that familiar tingle in his loins. "Well, you still can.... Kiss me, that is," Matt replied.

The ice queen smiled and said slyly, "We'll see, but right now, you should go talk to the nurse so you can get your meds schedule. Everybody here is on a schedule. Come on, I'll show you." She turned and started walking down the hall. Matt followed close behind, admiring the way her booty moved rhythmically under her robe.

They came to a large common area with couches, tables for eating, and a large-screen television in one corner of the room. Matt watched the other patients in the ward who were milling about. One young man was pacing back and forth in front of the glass-walled nurse's station. Every couple of minutes, he'd knock on the glass to ask if it was time for his medication. Every time, the head nurse would say, "Not yet Robert. You still have a few hours before your night meds." Undeterred, Robert would be right back, two minutes later, and ask the same question. 'At least he's consistent,' Matt thought.

After getting his meds schedule from the nurse, Matt sat down next to the queen on one of the couches. He was determined to impress this girl, but first, he wanted to know more about her. "So, do you come here often?" he said jokingly.

"Actually, this is my second time here. My parents put me in here because they say I'm incorrigible, but I think it's because they're afraid of me," she said.

"Afraid of you? Why would they be afraid of you?" Matt asked.

She didn't hesitate when she said, "I threatened to burn the house down with them in it. Looking back, that probably wasn't too smart." Wow! Matt was beside himself. Beautiful and dangerous! He knew more than ever that he wanted this girl. 'I don't know how yet, but I've got two days to figure it out,' he thought.

Over the next twenty-four hours, Matt poured on the charm. He found out her name was Alicia, and the more he showed how attentive of a listener he was, the more she talked. She was twenty-five years old and lived with her parents in North Olmsted, after a break-up with her fiancé. "I caught him cheating with my best friend, so I got a gun, and if it wasn't for the gun misfiring, I would have shot them both," Alicia said, without a bit of remorse. Her parents pulled some strings with the judge when she went to court. The jail time would be suspended as long as she submitted to a psyche evaluation. Thus, her first visit to St. Vincent.

"Now that I'm on paper, my folks can have me probated just by saying 'she threatened to kill us,'" she said matter-of-factly.

"I guess saying you'd burn the house down with them in it would qualify," Matt agreed. As they talked more, Matt was becoming enthralled by this strange, beautiful woman. Her outgoing personality was refreshing to him, and the way she would lightly touch his arm when she laughed at something funny he said sent shivers through his body.

She told him she used to be a model for department stores all across Ohio when she was a teenager. The rift between Alicia and her parents came when she told them she wanted to model professionally. "My father hit the ceiling," she remembered. "He wanted me to go to law school and join his firm. I had no interest in becoming a lawyer. It's too boring... just like my father!" Matt spent the rest of the day, and all of the next, getting to know Alicia better. She seemed to be just as interested in him as he was in her. She even went so far as to give him a kiss on the cheek when he got the nurse to give him a before-bedtime snack, because Alicia said she was still hungry after dinner. "I see you have the powers of persuasion with the nurses, Mr. Green," she said coyly. Matt did something totally out of his character. He started blushing.

"Always willing to help a damsel in distress," he said.

By the start of the fourth day of his hospitalization, Matt was worried he wouldn't get his chance with Alicia. She was becoming more touchy-feely with him, frequently giving him hugs, and once, a kiss on the lips. However, with the nursing staff keeping a close watch on them, he knew it would be next to impossible to get her alone. But he wasn't giving up just yet.

After dinner that day, Alicia said to Matt, "Under other circumstances, I believe we would be an item."

Matt was feeling bold, and a little desperate, when he said, "We could still be an item, right here, right now. We probably won't see each other again after tomorrow, so we should make the best of our time while we can."

Alicia's eyes lit up, and she leaned in close to whisper in his ear. "You know, you're right. After we get our night meds, come to my room." She then gave him a playful nibble on his ear, which sent shock waves through him, and walked back to her room to "take a nap and get ready for later."

The hours leading up to the dispensing of their night meds seemed interminable to Matt. All he could think about was Alicia and her invitation to come to her room. He hadn't seen her since she'd gone to take a nap, but he knew she would be waiting for him later. He hadn't devised a plan for what he had in mind, but he was willing to let things develop spontaneously. Besides, it was her idea. Maybe she already has a plan. He was anxious to find out.

By 10 p.m., the meds had been all handed out, and the nurses began to relax, knowing the patients would be asleep for the night.

The following is a description of what transpired from Matt's notebook journal:

"I caught the nurses off guard and walked casually down the hall toward my room. Alicia's room was next to mine, so I passed up my room to walk by hers. Her door was partially opened, and I could see her standing naked with her back to me. I slipped quietly into her room, closing the door behind me. We fell into each other's arms, kissing passionately, and feverishly pulling down my pajama bottoms. We enjoyed all of three minutes of sex before one of the nurses burst in and broke up our tryst."

Even though they were interrupted, both Alicia and Matt felt they had thumbed their noses at the system in the ultimate fashion. They had managed a brief sexual encounter in the psyche ward of St. Vincent Charity Hospital, something that was totally forbidden. To them, there could be no finer way to say "fuck the establishment."

However, as Matt predicted, this was the last time he'd see Alicia. Because of their "extreme violation" of hospital rules, Matt was sent back to his room, but Alicia was put into "temporary seclusion," a term used for patients who needed to be watched constantly all day. By morning, she had been transferred to another facility.

A day later, Matt was discharged. He felt great, and with it being late October, he was looking forward to the coming holiday season.

The year 2007 ended on a happy note for Matt, but the coming year would prove to be even more challenging for him personally. Not to mention, tragic.

CHAPTER 19

The Dark Year

"Come my love, let's have big fun. Let's dance and frolic under the sun. But let's be quick, we must move fast. They say that nothing good will ever last."

A poem by Matt Green

Matt started 2008 with high hopes and expectations. He admitted to himself the previous year had been fun, but unproductive.

"I don't know exactly what to think of 2007," he wrote in his notebook journal dated "New Year's Day, 2008." "It was kind of spent in a blur. My only wish for this year is higher productivity, on all fronts."

Initially, he was on that path. He turned twenty-one that year, and knew he had to start doing things differently. He was taking his medication as prescribed, thus keeping his manic mood swings in check. He'd also started getting into his music again. I would hear him playing his acoustic and singing words to new songs he'd written, often into the late hours of the evening.

One day, after one of his lengthy practice sessions, I asked him, "Have you found a new girlfriend or something? I haven't heard you practice this much since the Gypsy Gibsons."

He just smiled and said, "No, nothing like that. I just know I'm not going to be a famous rock star, but I can still make music that could make a difference." He told me his buddy Joe Revay was about to attend a music engineering school in Arizona, and he wanted him to be the producer of his new music. "I'm going to visit him this spring. I've saved some money, and I'm gonna fly out there. I can't wait!"

Even his interactions with Lynda and I were less confrontational. We hadn't had any arguments about his behavior, and I attributed that to his newfound interest in being healthy and complying with his doctor's orders. His whole demeanor had changed. He went from the brash, egotistical kid that thought he knew everything, to a more mature, introspective man. Lynda and I were cautiously optimistic; we'd been through too many of his episodes to totally relax. However, we never showed him anything but encouragement and love.

He was still smoking marijuana, which worried me somewhat. I couldn't be sure if that would trigger another episode, but all it seemed to do was make him more amenable, so I didn't make a fuss about it. He began reading eastern philosophy, and was becoming fascinated with spirituality, something he'd never shown an interest in before. "I want to know more about the soul, the essence of man."

I have to say, I was proud of the change in attitude Matt was exhibiting. I'd never seen him so confident and thriving in his fledgling manhood. "This is gonna be a great year for me, dad. I just know it!" he said as he boarded the plane to Arizona to see Joe. It was his first time traveling on his own, and he couldn't be more excited.

The first few months of the year went without incident. He came back from his time in Arizona well rested and happier than I'd seen him in a long time. Lynda and I were ecstatic that Matt seemed to be ready to take responsibility for his health and well-being. I was very happy for him, and proud too.

Then in April of that year, the peaceful existence of the previous months was about to come to an end. After a routine colonoscopy, Lynda was informed by her doctor a polyp was removed from her colon. A subsequent biopsy found it to be cancerous. My beautiful, fun-loving wife had colon cancer. The news was devastating to the family, but to Matt especially.

"Dad, is mom gonna die?" he asked. I could see the anxiety on his face.

"No, Matt. The doctor said because it was detected early, and it hasn't spread, she should be fine after surgery to remove the section where the polyp was located."

I could see he wasn't totally convinced, but all he said was, "I'm going to my room. I need to think awhile." I was worried about Lynda of course, but at that moment, I was more concerned about Matt. I didn't know if this would be a reason for him to stop the progress he'd been making and revert to his old behavior. I knew he wasn't one to show much emotion, but I knew how close of a relationship he had with his mother. He would not be able to handle life without her.

Two weeks after the initial diagnosis, Lynda had surgery to remove the affected section of colon. The surgery was successful, and she recovered amazingly fast. However, I noticed a subtle change in Matt afterward. He started spending more time in his room, some days not coming out at all. His usual loquaciousness became short, monotone sentences. I continued watching him closely to make sure he was still keeping up with his meds. I was also looking for any signs he wasn't sleeping, which was a sure indicator he was on the verge of another manic episode. However, he seemed more determined than ever to stay on the straight and narrow.

When I asked him if he was still worried about his mother, he said, "I'm okay. She's doing fine so far, and I know she's got the whole family praying for her. I don't want her to have more problems worrying about me." Then he said, "And don't you worry either. I'm not gonna mess up again. I promise."

True to his word, Matt stuck to his routine. He continued writing music, and was attentive to Lynda's needs during her convalescence. I did notice he started reading more about the supernatural, and topics dealing with near-death experiences. Other than this new morbid (I thought) curiosity, he seemed to be getting over the crisis the family had gone through.

Slowly, our household got back to normal. Follow up visits to the doctor showed no recurrence of the cancer, but Lynda would have to have yearly screenings for the next five years. "If nothing shows up in that time, you can consider yourself cancer-free" he told us.

Three months later came another blow. On July 23rd, 2008, my sister, Rosa Ann Sloan, died after accidentally falling from the third floor balcony of her daughter's apartment. She was fifty-eight years old. Rosa was one of Matt's favorite aunts. She would always give him praises when he played his guitar for her, and he identified with her outgoing nature and her refusal to be dictated to. Questioning authority was in her DNA, and she did it whenever she felt it was necessary. She delighted in making people uneasy, and didn't mind arguing with anyone who didn't agree with her free-wheeling approach to life.

To Matt, she was the epitome of the non-conformist he thought himself to be, and he loved her dearly for it. He also felt, to some degree, she actually understood him. "I'm like Auntie Rosa in a way. She told me not to take shit from anybody, and I don't either. I'm gonna miss her, dad."

"Me too, son, me too," I said and gave him a hug. He went to his room, and for the next few days, hardly came out. I was afraid he was going into a depression, but then I'd hear him playing his guitar, and thought he was just coping with her death the best way he knew how... through his music.

After Rosa's funeral (he was quiet through the whole service), Matt showed an even keener interest in mysticism and the hereafter. He got tarot cards and started reading books on how to interpret them. He studied numerology, and astrology, as well as books on occultism. Creepy, I thought, but as long as he was taking better care of himself, who was I to question his reading material?

Again, things were going pretty well for us. We were still keeping a watchful eye on Matt, but just two months after his aunt's untimely death, he would get even more devastating news.

His close childhood friend since moving to Bedford, and former Gypsy Gibsons bandmate, Eric Harms, passed away in the fall of that year. He was twenty-two years old. Matt was inconsolable. "What's happening dad? Why is this turning out to be such a messed up year? I thought this was going to be a good year for me, and it's turning out to be the worst year ever!"

I'd never seen him so upset before. I felt helpless, unable to give him an adequate answer. All I could come up with was, "I don't know what to say, Matt. Unfortunate things sometimes happen to good people. There's no explanation for it. That's just the way life is. No one said it was fair. We just have to deal with tragedy the best way we can, and move on." That sounded lame even to me, but that was all I could come up with.

"I want to go to the funeral. Will you go too?" he asked with utter sadness in his eyes.

"Of course I'll go. Lynda will too. You know we all loved Eric."

"Thanks" was all he said, and went to his room, which by now, I considered his sanctuary.

A few days later, when we got to the funeral home for the viewing, Matt got out of the car so fast I hadn't even put the car in park. Lynda and I followed, and while we were talking with the family, Matt was already in the main chapel looking down at his friend in a beautifully ornate casket. His back was to us so I couldn't see his face, but Eric's brother, Greg Slawinski, was standing next to him with an arm around his shoulder.

"When I called Matt to tell him Eric died, all he said was 'wow!' He didn't sound like he was surprised at all. But when he actually saw Eric, he started crying immediately. I knew then he was taking it pretty hard, because I'd never seen Matt cry before…. ever."

Lynda and I barely had time to pay our respects when Matt grabbed my arm and said, "Can we leave now dad? I don't want to be here anymore." I was a little surprised by his request.

"Don't you want to stay for the service?"

"I can't do it. I can't stay. Can we go please?" I could see the anguish on his face. His eyes were already red from the tears he'd cried, and from the ones he was trying hard to hold back. "Okay, Matt. We can leave," and just as abruptly as we came, we left.

There seemed to be a marked difference in him after that. He became more stoic, and secretive. His mood changed, although it wasn't the same as the mood swings of an episode. It was more of a brooding nature, as if he were constantly in a funk.

It apparently affected the others in his close circle of friends. "There was a big shift when Eric died," said Sarah Solomon. "We spent a lot more time together, but there was way too much drinking going on too."

However, there was some good that came from Eric's passing. Matt and Jesse Carter, who hadn't spoken for the previous three years since their fight outside Peabody's, finally reconciled their differences. "We actually had a jam session and played some of the old Gypsy Gibson songs," Jesse remembered. "It felt good to jam with Matt again, but it was sort of weird because Eric wasn't there."

To his credit, I could see Matt was trying hard to keep focused on his health. He was still keeping his doctor's appointments and taking his meds, but something was different. He didn't have the same enthusiasm he'd displayed earlier in the year, which I totally understood. I wasn't worried yet, but I was concerned about his mental state. He wasn't talking to us about how he felt. Even when asked, he'd only say "I'm okay. You don't have to keep asking me that." All we could do was stay vigilant.

"Please God," I prayed one night. "Don't let anything more happen. We can't handle any more bad news."

Not even two months later, God showed me he had a cruel sense of humor. After a routine physical, my doctor said he believed I had an enlarged prostate. More testing would be needed, but he said African American men of my age (54) were more prone to the condition, but I shouldn't be too alarmed. "But as a precaution, I'm ordering a biopsy on the tissue to make sure it isn't anything more serious.

Well guess what? It was. The results from the biopsy confirmed I had prostate cancer. As the great Alan Freed used to say, "The hits just keep on comin'!" However, as in Lynda's case, because it was detected early, the doctor was relatively sure I could beat it. "We'll start treatment immediately, and hopefully the cancer can be arrested," he said. Hell yeah, arrest that bastard, I thought to myself.

Of course, this brought another heavy pall upon our house. Upon hearing the news, Matt went into a deeper depressive state. My assurances I was going to be fine after treatment didn't help at all. He started writing sad poems, and the music he played had a dark tone. He wouldn't hold eye contact for more than a few minutes, and when he'd talk, he always seemed distracted.

As it turned out, my radiosurgery was a success. A new technology called the Cyberknife was used to precisely target my prostate, and using lasers, eradicated the cancerous tissue that was there. Like Lynda, I'd have to have yearly screenings for the next five years, to make sure there was no recurrence, but other than that, the doctor said I should be fine.

I thought the good news would bring Matt out of his melancholy, but it didn't. He continued being mostly quiet, and even irritable. He would get upset whenever I'd ask how he was feeling. "I keep telling you I'm fine. Why don't you believe me?"

He wrote in his journal in bold caps, "DAD THINKS WAY TOO MUCH! CARES WAY TOO MUCH!" If he only knew how true those words were.

The holiday season of 2008 brought very little joy to the Green household. What started out as year of eagerly awaited good fortune turned into a year of dark despair. I, for one, was glad to see it come to an end, but with Matt, I was wary of when the other shoe was going to drop.

CHAPTER 20

The Green Fairy

"The choice to consume alcohol was a rite of passage to me, and it's one that I took seriously too".

-Matt Green-

The following year began without incident. Matt was still taking his meds on schedule, and making all his appointments with his doctors. Since he was now getting a monthly disability check, he was able to buy the clothes he felt were befitting of his new attitude.

He was already an avid reader of GQ magazine, but now he was ordering shirts and coats online that were fitted to flatter his tall, slender frame. He called it being the "Modern Gentleman," and wanted to be more refined in his attire.

I had to admit he was looking quite handsome as he was now sporting a nicely rounded Afro, with a full beard and mustache. His brother John had gotten his barber's license, and he was the only one Matt would allow to cut his hair, or shape his beard. After spending an hour in John's barber chair, Matt would come home looking like one of the models he admired in GQ.

He was very conscious of his appearance, and knew the affect it had on women. "I know I look good," he said once as he modeled his new fitted shirt, vest, and skinny jeans. "But wait 'til they see me now!" It seemed the malaise that had been with him for most of the previous year had finally let go. He was back to being his jovial, confident, yet goofy self, and Lynda and I took notice.

In the spring of the year, he said, "Hey dad, guess what? I got financial aid for college. I'm going to enroll at Tri-C and take real estate classes!" He was so excited he'd done this on his own, without our help. "I'm gonna get into the real estate market and make a lot of money. What do you think?"

I was as happy as he was, but not for the same reason. Secretly, I was afraid on any given day, he'd stop taking his meds and become sick again. With this revelation, I felt he'd actually turned the corner toward better health.

"That's great, Matt. When will you start?"

"I've just gotten a confirmation on my FASFA application, so I can start in the summer semester. I can't wait!" Once again, I was overjoyed for Matt. He seemed to be on the right track, and he also appeared to be determined to work hard to accomplish his real estate goal. There had been no episodes in over a year, so I kept my fingers crossed that there wouldn't be another any time soon. I wasn't naïve to think he was cured of his bipolar disorder; there is no cure. However, I felt at least with him managing himself better, any recurring episodes wouldn't be so severe.

In the weeks leading up to his enrollment at Tri-C, Matt got as many books from the library about real estate investments as they would allow. He read every one, returned them, and always came back with more. He would eagerly describe to Lynda and I how the short sales, foreclosures, and note purchasing were all lucrative ways to make money in the market. His enthusiasm was contagious, and for a little while, he had me reading some of his books too. I could see how real estate could make a ton of money, but I also knew it would take a ton of commitment to make it work. I had no doubt Matt had the determination, but like anything he was really interested in, he would become obsessed to the point of exhaustion. This would lead him to do things to stay up that were not necessarily good for his health.

Late one night, as I was heading to the bathroom to relieve my two-cent bladder, I saw a light coming from under the door of Matt's room. Because it was 3 a.m., I was wondering if he'd left his television on and fallen asleep, something he'd frequently done after taking his night meds.

I opened his door quietly, not wanting to wake him up. To my surprise, he was not only awake, but reading a book while sipping on some green liquid in a small, funny-shaped glass. He looked up at me, and with a smile said, "What's up dad?" as if it were the middle of the day.

"Apparently you still are." I immediately reflected back on his previous episodes, all of which began with him staying up late and not sleeping. "Did you take your night meds?"

"Yeah dad, I always do," he said dismissively. Then he lightened up and said, "Hey dad, this book is great. It's called 'Protecting Your #1 Asset."

I wasn't thinking about the book. I wanted to know what he was drinking, so I asked him, "What's that," pointing to the glass with the mysterious green liquid. He must have thought I was asking about his book because he replied, "According to the author, our number one asset is our intellectual property. I could create a fortune turning my ideas into assets. That's a brilliant concept. I wish I'd thought of it."

"No Matt, what's in the glass?"

He looked at the glass admiringly and said, "Oh this? This is 'La Fee Verte.'"

Confused, I replied, "What did you say?"

He answered condescendingly, "That's French, dad. It means the 'Green Fairy.'" Now, my mind was thinking all kinds of irrational thoughts.

"The green what?"

"The Green Fairy. That's what they call absinthe."

Absinthe. Originating in Switzerland in the 1800s, it

became popular among the artists and writers of that era. I'd heard of the spirit before, but all I really knew was it was banned in the United States in the early 1900s. I knew writers like Earnest Hemingway and James Joyce, as well as artists like Vincent Van Gogh and Pablo Picasso consumed it. I also heard it had hallucinogenic properties, something I didn't think Matt needed right now.

"Do you think it's wise to be drinking that stuff while you're on medication?" I was trying to be diplomatic. I didn't want him to think I was going to nag him about it. From past experience, that would be the easiest way to make him do more of what I wanted him to stop doing.

"Don't worry. It's only a couple of ounces, and I'm not drinking it, I'm *sipping* it. There is a distinct difference, you know."

Continuing in my diplomatic role, I said, "But isn't absinthe supposed to make you hallucinate?" He laughed,

"That's a myth everybody believes. It does have a high alcohol content, but that's why you only have a little at a time, and sip it slowly. I've been tasting on it for the past couple of weeks, and I haven't had one hallucination." Then he said, almost to himself, "I was hoping I would, though."

Two weeks? I was flabbergasted. If he'd been drinking... sorry, sipping that stuff for that long without us knowing, what else was he doing in secret that might be harmful to his health? To keep him from sipping anymore, I said, "Let me try it."

He got a big grin on his face and said, "I knew you'd want to try it. I'll fix you one of your own."

He reached in a drawer next to his bed and pulled out a wooden box. Inside was a green bottle with "Pernod" on the label. There was another glass like the one he had, and a funny-shaped spoon fitted in the protective foam padding. In a small silk pouch, he had a few sugar cubes.

"What's all that, Matt?" Now I was getting curious.

"Don't touch anything. I have to get some more ice water." He grabbed a small plastic water pitcher (ironically taken from his last hospital stay), and rushed to the kitchen. I could hear him getting ice from the trays in the freezer, and he came back in record time with the pitcher filled with ice and a bottle of water. I hadn't seen him this happy since we had our first beer together.

"Here dad," he said as he handed me the pitcher. "Pour about half that bottle of water in the pitcher. I'm going to fix it the way it was originally done. It's an art to it." Dutifully, I did as I was told and watched as he sat the glass on top of the book he'd been reading. I noticed the glass had a bulbous bottom that flared out at the top. He then gently lifted the Pernod from its padding, uncorked the top, and carefully poured the clear greenish liquid into the glass, being sure not to overfill past the bulbous bottom.

Next, he took the spoon and placed it on top of the glass.

For the first time, I saw the intricate designs cut into the bowl of the spoon, and small hooks on the side to hold it in place. He reached in the pouch and pulled out a single sugar cube, placing it gently on the spoon. Still staring intently at his creation, he reached out his hand and said, "Okay dad, let me have the pitcher." He had the look of pure concentration on his face, and like a scientist in a lab, he leaned over the glass and said, "Now watch what happens when I add water. You're gonna like this part."

I watched, transfixed as he ever so slowly poured the ice water over the sugar cube. He was doing it so slowly, the water seemed to be dripping rather than pouring out. The designs cut into the spoon allowed the water and dissolving sugar to leech into the glass. As the mixture hit the absinthe, I could see the once clear liquid slowly turn opaque. "See that, dad? It's called the louche affect."

He poured only a few ounces of water onto the sugar cube before it was completely dissolved, but it seemed like it took an hour for him to do it. I was somewhat mesmerized not only by Matt's theatrics, but by the seemingly magical way the clear liquid turned a cloudy green.

"Ok Matt, now what?" I said impatiently. The whole ritual took about ten minutes, and I was more than ready to try out this forbidden elixir. He could see my eagerness and decided to make me wait a little longer. "

Just a second, dad. You can't rush greatness." He swirled

the mixture a few times, lifted the glass to his nose and took a sniff. "Ah, now it's ready. Here you go, dad. Let me introduce you to La Fee Verte, the Green Fairy." With a flourish he hands me the glass.

I had to give it to him. His presentation was flawless, and I was totally hooked. Rather than being the responsible one, warning him about the dangers of drinking alcohol while on medication, here I was ready to do exactly what he wanted me to do... drink with him. Some parent I was.

I felt as if I were about to go on a journey of strangeness, and he was my guide. All the things I'd heard about the hazards of consuming absinthe, were erased from my mind. All I was thinking was, I'm about to have the drink of famous artists and writers. I'm about to feel what they felt.

With great anticipation, I took a small sip. Once the viscous liquid reached my taste buds, I was slammed back into reality. Let me say, I've never liked sweets of any kind. I don't eat cake, pies, or pastry. My sweet tooth must have been pulled at a very early age, because I didn't like to go trick-or-treating on Halloween because all I ever got was candy. YUK!

The taste of this absinthe was not only sweet, but it reminded me of the worse candy I'd ever tasted... black licorice! I almost gagged.

Matt was in hysterics. He knew all along I wouldn't like it, but he reeled me in like a complete sucker. "You should see the look on your face, dad. It's priceless!" He was in tears from laughing so hard. Now, I was really pissed. Just so he could see I was no wimp, I gulped down the entire glass of the awful stuff. Matt stopped laughing and got a serious look on his face. "Oh shit, dad, you shouldn't have done that. That stuff is 160 proof. You're gonna be sick."

Still being macho, I say, "It's nasty, but I've drank plenty of nasty liquor before. I'm not gonna get sick," and I stormed out of his room. Well needless to say, he was right. I spent the rest of that night tossing and turning with a feeling of an imminent upheaval. My stomach was churning, and I eventually had to throw up the Green Fairy. Once the vile concoction was safely in the toilet, and out of my stomach, I felt a little better. I gladly flushed that bitch down the plumbing.

By morning, I had the worst hangover I'd had in a long time. As I sat at the kitchen table nursing a cup of strong coffee (black, NO sugar!), Matt came down all bright-eyed, ready for school. He sat across from me and just looked with a grin on his face.

"Don't say a word," I warn. "I'm not in the mood". Just then his ride blew the horn in the driveway.

He got up, slapped me on the back and said, "Don't worry dad, you'll get used to it. Remember, 'you've had plenty of nasty tasting liquor before.'" Then he hurriedly ran out the door before I could cuss his ass out.

CHAPTER 21

Matt and Molly

School for Matt was enjoyable. He'd always found classes easy to pass all through his education. However, the more intense challenge of college was more to his liking.

"High school was too easy," he said once. "The criteria to be successful in college will require me to stay focused. I can't just go through the motions anymore." His grades proved he was staying focused. He had straight 'A's in his real estate classes, and he'd also gotten 'A's in his philosophy class, something I had no idea he was taking.

"I consider myself a philosopher too, dad. I'm not just a musician or a capitalist. Both have to be driven by some sort of philosophy. That's why I took the class." His determination to do well in school was admirable, but I knew, for him, he needed to balance things with some form of relaxation. All work and no play could cause Matt to have another episode. So I asked him if he was doing anything other than study for entertainment.

"I've been hanging out with a 'friend' for a while, and we've been keeping each other occupied," He said in his now familiarly cryptic fashion. I took from that he was seeing a girl. He'd never admit it, but I knew that was the case.

After the first semester was completed and he'd registered for the fall, I started noticing a shiny red car dropping him off, and on occasion, picking him up. He'd never say who the mystery person was. He'd bound out of the house before we could make any inquiries. I told Lynda my theory, and as mothers do, she did a little more investigating. "I don't know her name yet, but I'll get it." Matt was about to be confronted.

One morning when the red car pulled up, she corralled him before he could leave. "Who's that girl, Matt? Is she your girlfriend?" Lynda didn't mince words when she wanted information.

"No mom, we're just friends. Her name is Molly Matosky. She's the one who's been giving me rides." Then he said, "Well, I gotta go," and rushed from the house. We both watched from the window as he got in her car, gave her a quick peck on the cheek, and they drove off. We looked at each other, both of us thinking the same thing, but Lynda voicing it.

"Matt has a girlfriend. I don't care what he says."

Throughout his life, Matt was pretty predictable. He'd

spend most of his free time reading, or hanging out with his friends. For the previous two years, he and Tom were almost inseparable. They would get together first thing in the morning, and wouldn't get home until late in the evening.

"I'd call Matt, then drive into Bedford to pick him up. Some days, we would be at the Bedford Ledges playing music and talking about philosophy on the rocks. Other days would find us in Lakewood, or Cleveland, playing an acoustic show at a coffee shop," Tom remembered. "We had a lot of fun back then."

By the fall of 2009, Matt was spending most of his time with Molly. Her red car would pull up, and by now, she wasn't just waiting in her car for him to come out. She'd come in and talk to Lynda and I while waiting for him to get ready. She was a cute girl, with longish dark hair that shined a little when under direct light. She had expressive eyes and a crooked smile that I found somewhat endearing. You could tell she really liked Matt because when he came in the room, that smile would immediately come on her face, and there was no mistaking the admiring look in her eyes.

Although in front of us, Matt would try to come across as stoic and unemotional, we could see he really liked her too by the way his face lit up when he saw her. Lynda and I knew they were both quite taken with each other. As Melissa Deal, one of his closest female friends would put it, "He loved her a lot. A lot, a lot, a lot! During their relationship, he and I weren't allowed to be friends. He was very straight forward about that."

Matt had essentially cut off his longtime friends so he could spend more time with Molly, and it was a positive thing for him. Initially, their relationship appeared to be the calming influence that he needed in his life. However, we started to notice Matt staying up later and later toward the end of 2009. We would hear him patrolling the house, going up and down the stairs, well beyond the time he should have been asleep. We attributed it to school having started, and he was probably wound up from studying. He hadn't had an episode in over a year by this time, so we were willing to give him the benefit of the doubt.

By October, there was no change in his behavior, but we did notice his agitation when he spoke about Molly. "We had an argument," he said when I asked him about her. "She's so jealous sometimes, and accuses me of cheating on her." Sometimes, I would see scratches on his arms, and when I'd ask him about them, all he'd say was, "She did it."

"Listen Matt, if you two are starting to have fights, maybe it's time for you to take a break." He wouldn't hear of it.

"Don't worry, dad. I can handle it."

His not sleeping at night hadn't stopped for a few weeks, and I was starting to be concerned. "Are you taking your meds like you're supposed to, Matt? I've noticed you haven't been sleeping much lately." He gave me that dismissive look of his when he doesn't want to be bothered.

"I've been taking my meds, but I've been trying to work on my real estate deals, and that's causing me to stay up late to make phone calls."

"Who would you be calling at 2 or 3 o'clock in the morning Matt?"

"The people I'm talking about live on the west coast, so it's only 11 or 12 o'clock at night there. Come on dad, don't bug me about it." That was it. I no longer believed he was taking his meds, and I was convinced he was on the verge of another manic episode. I watched him closely for the next few days and saw how he would pace the floor like a caged animal, all the while talking rapidly about the lucrative real estate deals he was hatching.

Sometimes, I could hear him talking loudly on the phone, presumably to Molly, in an authoritative voice, ending the call with, "Just come by and pick me up!" I saw the worried look on her face when she came to the house. I went out to her car before Matt came out to talk to her. "Molly, we have to put up with Matt because we're his parents, but you don't have to. Are you sure you're okay with Matt? I know how hard it can be sometimes when he's not himself."

She gave me a sad look but said, "It's okay, Mr. Green. I've seen him this way before and I can usually calm him down. He just gets agitated easily sometimes, but we'll be alright."

I felt for her at that moment and wondered how long it

would be before she tired of his mood swings. "Alright Molly. Just remember what I said." Just then, Matt came bounding out of the house and into her passenger seat.

"Let's go," he said, and they pulled out of the driveway. Shortly after that, Matt had to be hospitalized.

There was some incident that happened at Tri-C, and he had to be escorted off the campus by security. When I went to pick him up, his eyes were wide, and he couldn't stop talking incessantly about how his rights had been violated. "Those fuckers kicked me out of class because I told the teacher he didn't know what he was talking about." I tried to make sense of the situation so I pressed on.

"Is that all, Matt? What else happened?" He seemed glad I asked that question because he immediately answered, and what he said next let me know where I had to take him.

"I told him I knew more about real estate than he did, and that I'd teach the class. When I went up front to do it, he called security!" He said it as if he had every right to teach that class.

Needless to say, he was at Marymount Hospital's psychiatric ward once again, this time for a week. Even after his discharge, I could tell he wasn't one hundred percent well. He still had these grand ideas about real estate and how he was going to make millions. All the while, Molly stuck by his side. They would have frequent arguments, but somehow they'd always manage to stay together. I felt sorry for her knowing how trying Matt could be, but I knew when she'd had enough, she would cut him loose. As she would tell me later, "Matt was becoming more and more irritable, and we'd have arguments more frequently. I even suggested we end the relationship a couple of times, but he didn't want to talk about it."

The events of April 25, 2010 would be the end of the relationship... for good. That day, Molly picked up Matt right after working out at the gym. By this time, Matt was once again in a manic state, and his emotions were amplified. 'I know she wasn't at the gym. She was with another guy,' he thought, and he intended to let her know it.

"He started right in on me," Molly would later say, "Telling me I wasn't at the gym, and getting really agitated." She'd had enough and told him she was going to take him home.

"No, no," he protested, "I'll be alright." However, he wouldn't stop his accusations.

Molly decided to take him to her house because she needed to take a shower. While there, she told him to wait in the living room until she finished. By this time, Matt's mind was racing. He just knew she was cheating on him, and the thought of that incensed him. He wasn't going to sit there and wait for her to wash that other guy's scent off. He was going in there and catch her before she did.

"I was undressed and about to get in the shower, and Matt breaks down my bathroom door." She starts screaming at him to get out, but Matt wasn't hearing it. He just started taking off his clothes. "I think he wanted to get in the shower with me," she said, "But I knew he wasn't in his right mind, which scared me. I didn't know what he was going to do. It was really scary."

She put her clothes back on with the intention of taking him home, but Matt had other ideas. "He'd put the couch in front of the front door, and he took my keys from me and locked the dead bolt on the back door. He took my cell phone, and we started pushing and shoving each other," she remembered. Matt finally pinned her to the floor, with her screaming for him to get off her, but he wouldn't let her up. "I wasn't angry at him about it because I knew he was bipolar, but it was just so sad."

She eventually got away long enough to make a quick call to 911 on the fax machine she had in her house. She waited until she heard someone answer before hanging up. "Matt grabs me again and "chokes me out. After that, I felt defeated." Molly relented and let Matt get her into the shower with him. Suddenly, she heard her dog barking loudly, and the next thing she knew, "the police had broken down the door and had their guns out. They found us naked in the shower." Then, that crooked smile came on her face when she said, "It was epic!"

Matt was taken to the Bedford jail again and charged with assault and unlawful restraint. By this time, he was in a full-on manic episode and wouldn't comply with the booking officer. I went to see him, after a call from the police, and he wouldn't even talk to me. He just stared blankly, his eyes moving rapidly back and forth. I was totally frustrated with Matt and told the officer to do what they had to do. Lynda and I had had enough of Matt and his antics. We decided to let the courts handle him, and let his actions dictate his future.

He was a twenty-three-year-old man who could no longer avoid the consequences of his indiscretions. As much as it hurt us, we had no choice but to make that decision.

CHAPTER 22

Scary Matt

"Fools call me crazy, insane, and plain dumb. I like them."

-Matt Green-

After his breakup with Molly, Matt couldn't seem to get his shit together. He went around the house as if in a daze. He spent a lot of time in his room, either playing sad songs on his guitar, or reading. Because of the "shower incident," he was convicted of disorderly conduct, and since he hadn't been going to his court appearances, he was also convicted of contempt of court. He was on "paper," having to report to his probation officer once a week. He was taking his medication (also a requirement of his probation), but only sparingly, which caused Lynda and I to always be on edge.

He wasn't drinking as much, but he was still smoking weed. In fact, even though he was on probation, and subject to urine testing, he wouldn't stop. I was sitting in the office when his probation officer told Matt he'd be tested regularly for drugs. "You might as well lock me up now, 'cause I'm gonna come up dirty." I was flabbergasted at Matt's brazenness, waiting for the officer's reaction. All he said was, "Okay, Matthew, just make sure you call me every Friday to report in. I won't test you as long as you call in. But if you miss just one call while still on probation, I'm bringing you in for a test. If you come up positive for drugs of any kind, I'll have your ass locked up. Do you understand?"

Matt sat back in his seat and said smugly, "Yeah, I get it."

I couldn't believe what I was hearing. Matt had just told this guy he wasn't going to stop smoking while on probation, and all he said was don't miss a call or he'd be tested. That seemed to be typical of Matt when dealing with the judicial system. He'd fall in a pile of shit, and somehow, come out smelling like a rose.

He wasn't afraid of going to jail because, as he told his brother Eddie once, "If we were to get arrested, I wouldn't go to the same jail as you. They'd put me in a court-ordered hospital until I was well enough to go to court. I can do that standing on my head!"

He started writing poems about love and how he could never find it. He even started writing about whether he should let his "internal polarities" (read: bipolar disorder) take over his life. "I have so many pre-existing internal polarities that the question becomes, should I seek to balance them, or should I allow them free reign in my mind, for better or worse?"

He would try to control his episodes by experimenting with his medications. He wouldn't take his pills daily as prescribed. He would spend the days he didn't, smoking weed and drinking beer with his buddies. He claimed the marijuana helped stabilize his moods as much, or more than, his medication. Of course, I knew that was a cop-out, but there was no telling Matt he was, or even could be, wrong.

We could see when he was on the verge of an episode, but just when we thought it was imminent, he'd somehow calm himself down. Maybe he was right after all about the marijuana. However, Lynda and I still remained vigilant. Our history with Matt didn't give us much choice.

Over the months, we'd become used to his back and forth moods. Okay, he wasn't taking his meds as he should, and he was still drinking and smoking, but as long as he wasn't aggravating his mother and I, what was the harm?

However, although he wasn't giving us any immediate grief, his friends weren't that lucky. Matt's close circle of friends all knew of his mental illness, but they remained loyal to the end. However, when they encountered Matt while in the throes of that "annoying exhilaration," they'd be left in a bind, trying to explain his behavior to others.

As his longtime friend Melissa Deal said, "When he'd have an episode, he would make people very uncomfortable.

We couldn't see why he was acting the way he was. If we were out together, and someone got too close to me, he'd say, 'Don't talk to her,' and he'd threaten them if they did. He thought, for some reason, someone would try to harm me. He'd become overly protective of me at those times."

Over the years, I saw the episodes become more and more frequent, especially when he wasn't taking his meds as he should. Each time, the only way for him to get better was to do something to get admitted to a hospital. In a way, I started to wonder if he intentionally triggered his symptoms, just so he could get the necessary treatment he'd never admit he needed.

However, after each recurring episode, it was becoming harder for him to recover. The words of his first psychiatrist, Dr. Miller, came back to me. "If he continues to refuse to take his medication as he should, I'm afraid all I can do is be here to help you pick up the pieces." Since he hadn't been keeping his doctor appointments either, it was left to Lynda and I, and his friends, to pick those pieces up.

One day, he left the house in a full blown episode. I confronted him, and told him to stay home. "Matt, why don't you take your meds and stay home today? You can get a good night's sleep, and I'll take you to see the doctor tomorrow." As usual when he got this way, he felt he knew more than anybody else what was best for him.

"I'm not going to sit around waiting for you to get me

locked up" (his euphemism for hospitalized). "I'm leaving, and you can't stop me." He was right; I couldn't stop him, at least not without an altercation.

I knew he hadn't been sleeping and had stopped taking his meds altogether for more than two weeks. We would hear him walking back and forth in the hall outside our room in the middle of the night, sometimes talking to himself. This was very unnerving. I'd have to get up and persuade him to at least stay in his room so we could sleep. He'd oblige, but then he'd get on his cell phone and call his friends, usually Sam Sizemore.

"He'd call me in the middle of the night. At first, I couldn't tell anything was wrong. But after a few minutes of talking, I could tell he hadn't been taking his meds. He'd say stuff like, 'When I have my castle in Germany, you won't be able to come because you're a peasant.'" Sam would get so frustrated, he wouldn't continue the conversation with Matt.

"Dude, take your meds and get some sleep. When you get better, we'll go back to work on some music," he'd say, and then he would hang up.

As Matt was leaving the house, I heard him on his phone telling Greg Slawinski he was coming over. It never ceased to amaze me how Matt's episodes never cost him any of his close friendships. They were always loyal to him, and weathered the storm almost as much as we did. Never once had I seen them turn him away. I was very happy, and grateful, he had such good friends. However, at that moment, I felt for Greg because I knew, very shortly, there would be another test to their friendship.

"I'd just got off the phone with him, and he was knocking on my door in what seemed like five minutes," Greg remembered. Greg, Joe Revay, and Greg's brother Jason, were all at the house watching an Indian's game. When the knock on the door came, Jason looked out the window and said, "It's Matt, and he has a sword! Don't open the door!" According to Greg, that's when Jason and Joe made themselves scarce. "Joe hid behind the couch, and I don't know where Jason went. But I knew Matt wouldn't be carrying a sword, so I opened the door, slowly."

Greg saw Matt standing at the door, and looked down at his hands. He didn't have a sword, but he was holding a baseball bat. He must have picked it up in somebody's yard on the way over, Greg thought. "What's up Matt? Why are you carrying that bat?" Matt wouldn't say anything, only stared at him, his eyes moving rapidly back and forth. "I knew right away Matt wasn't himself, so I decided to let him in. I didn't want him getting in trouble with the cops."

Greg told Matt to come on in, but he'd have to leave the bat outside, which he did. The whole time, he hadn't said a word. Once in the house, Greg tried to act as if everything was okay, and that's when Jason and Joe came out of hiding to join them.

As Joe would tell me later, "The day before, he was alright, at least he seemed to be. But now here he was, acting weird. It was painful to watch, and scary too. You knew he was in there, but he wasn't showing."

Greg got Matt to sit down and watch the game. Then, he tried to get him talking. "Hey Matt, you want a piece of pizza?" He didn't respond. All he did was continue to stare at him. Greg was undeterred. He was determined to get his friend to acknowledge him. "I'll get you some pizza okay?" Still no response.

As Greg was getting the pizza, Joe and Jason sat uneasily, trying to watch the game but keeping a wary eye on Matt. Matt wasn't talking to them, only staring with those crazy eyes of his. Greg came in with the pizza on a plate and handed it to Matt. He looked at the pizza really hard, and then at Greg. "He grabs the pizza and throws it at me. He hit me right in the face with it," Greg told me.

"Matt, why did you do that?" Matt finally spoke, but what he was saying didn't make sense to them.

"He starts talking about Mongolians. That's his only point, the Mongolians. And then, he starts hitting himself and screaming," said Greg.

They eventually got him to settle down, but he wouldn't stay much longer, and left the house. He came home later that night, and I could tell he was worse off than when he left. "Matt, go up to your room. I'll be there in a minute so we can talk."

"Would you make me some tea first?" He sounded very tired. He always wanted Earl Grey tea when he was trying to fight his mania.

"Sure, Matt. Just go to your room and I'll be right up with your tea." I tried not to sound too concerned.

He slowly went up to his room, and I could see from his movements he was exhausted. I didn't know what he'd been up to. He'd been gone for several hours, but whatever it was, it wore him out. I quickly made his tea and went up to his room. He'd stripped down to his underwear and was lying on his bed.

"Here's your tea son." I handed him the steaming cup.

"Thanks, dad," was all he said. I sat at the edge of his bed and watched him drinking the tea. He closed his eyes as he sipped the tea, and for the first time, I noticed a small scratch on his forehead.

"How'd you get that scratch on your head?" He wouldn't answer, just kept drinking his tea. I didn't question him further. I knew from past experience he wouldn't talk until he was good and ready, especially during an episode.

He finished his tea, handed me the cup and said, "I'm pretty tired, dad. I really need some sleep. Would you close the door when you leave?" I was being dismissed.

"Okay, son. You get some sleep and we'll talk in the morning." I left his room thinking I would get a call from one of his friends soon, or worse yet, the police. I had no idea what his day was like while wandering the streets in that state of mind. I just prayed there would be no serious repercussions.

This was getting tiresome. Lynda and I loved our son dearly, but he was testing our patience to the limit. I didn't know how much more we could take.

CHAPTER 23

Here We Go Again

I'm feeling like a hole in the wall. What I once called void, I now call nothing at all. Maybe I've gone insane, or maybe I'm just enlightened. But it's all the same.

-Matt Green-

I never got any calls about Matt after his visit with Greg. He slept the entire day away, so we never got a chance to talk. When I did finally talk to him, it was only to ask him how he felt. "I feel like a dried up spitball underneath a desk in a public high school," he said, and then he chuckled a little. Well, I could see the sleep did him some good. I decided to press a little further. "Did you take your meds this morning?" The humorous moment left, and he got serious.

"I sure did, and I'm going to start taking them like I'm supposed to. I don't want another episode to hit me like this last one. It was brutal."

I was glad to hear him say it, but I also knew he'd eventually have a relapse. His patterns were set in stone. He'd start feeling better for a few good months, but because he was feeling better, he'd stop taking his meds, and the cycle would begin all over again. Oh well. I guess I shouldn't look a gift horse in the mouth... whatever that means.

Since the "incident" with Molly and their breakup, I noticed Matt's female friends were beginning to call him again. He had made it quite clear while he was in a relationship with her that they would have to stop contacting him. He mentioned she was jealous, and she didn't want him talking to any of his girl friends. He said he was not romantically inclined with any of them, that they were just good close friends, and I believed him. The girls in his inner circle were as loyal as the boys. However, they too would become frightened by his unpredictability when under the influence of a manic episode. Plus, the fact he was taller than most of his crowd, and those "scary eyes," had almost all of them on edge when he was not himself.

By Halloween of 2010, Matt had gone back to sporadically taking his meds. He was able to control his mood swings, barely, but he'd begun to smoke more weed, instead of taking the medicine. "I've found a few joints, and a few beers, are all I need to maintain a balance," he said. I wasn't about to let him get away with that statement, not after all we'd been through with him.

"Oh come on Matt. How can you honestly believe that? You know as well as I do, you have to take your meds." He wouldn't back down.

"I've been doing some experimenting, and I've found that marijuana does a better job of controlling my behavior." He was totally convinced he had the answer to his illness.

"You're the smartest dummy I know Matt," was all I could think to say.

Privately, I was more concerned with his alcohol consumption. I'd learned over the years that alcohol, more than marijuana, caused him to have episodes that eventually landed him in the hospital, or jail. I heard him say he was going to a local haunted house with some of his friends, and Melissa would be there soon to pick him up. I felt uneasy knowing there would be some drinking going on.

Later that evening, seemingly out of nowhere, Matt pulled out a half pint of brandy and said, "I need to get my mind right." Before I could stop him, he unscrewed the cap off the little bottle and took a good swig. "Ahh, that's what I'm talking about," he said. I didn't want him to finish the whole bottle, so I tried to get him to pass it to me. "Hey Matt, let me join you," I said, and reached out my hand for the liquor. "Okay," he said, and then he drained the rest of the bottle in two swallows.

"Sorry dad, too late." At that moment, I knew his night was going to end prematurely. He'd killed a half pint of eighty-proof brandy in less than ten minutes, and it was just a matter of time before he would feel the effects.

By the time Melissa came to pick him up, he was not only three-sheets-to-the-wind, but I could see he was on his way to a possible episode. His conversation was pressured, and he was talking rapidly about all the fun he was going to have at the haunted house. When Melissa came to pick him up, I could see she was eyeing Matt suspiciously, as if trying to gauge where he was coming from. Like all of his friends, she had seen him at his worse, but lately Matt had been able to cover up his behavior. At least enough to not worry them. However, with all of his over-the-top histrionics about the fun they were going to have, she probably had an idea something wasn't quite right.

Sure enough, about an hour after picking him up, Melissa brought him home. "He was talking a bunch of nonsense and being really aggressive toward people. He was in that 'being my protector' mode again. I had to bring him home," she remembered. He was still being belligerent when he got home, but I wasn't having any of it. I followed him to his room and told him I was through trying to help him. That I was going to let his own actions determine his fate.

"You're a grown man, Matt. It's time for you to be treated like one. If you get in trouble because you won't take better care of yourself, then so be it. I'm done with you and your behavior."

He gave me a drunken smile and said, "Good. That's what you should have done in the first place. I know how to take care of myself."

That was the last straw. Lynda and I made a vow to each other that Matt was not getting any more help from us. Let the chips fall where they may.

Following Halloween, and leading into the holiday season, Matt made a concerted effort to stay out of our way. He'd enrolled in the fall at Tri-C and was continuing to take his classes, but his inability to manage his illness took a toll on his grades. More than his grades, his bipolar symptoms, which he tried hard to control, were becoming more and more apparent. Finally, he got kicked out for a second time. "He followed a young lady all over campus and tried to talk to her. When he was rebuffed, he kept following her. She reported him to security, and when we tried to talk to him, he became aggressive toward us," said the campus policeman. "That's when we escorted him from school property. He's not allowed back, Mr. Green."

His disturbing behavior was causing even family members to be wary of him. Usually, during the holidays, we would have a house full of people coming over at any given time. However, by Christmas of 2010, he was totally manic. Family and friends were declining our invitations to visit. "He's become embarrassing," Lynda said to me.

Even Colleen Allison, one of Matt's closest friends, and

always in his corner, was staying away from him due to a frightening incident that happened at her house.

He'd come to her house "acting weird" one day, and when she went to her daughter's room to get something, he blocked the doorway so she couldn't get out. "I told him to get out of the way, that I wanted to leave the room, and he just stood there staring at me. It was scary," she said. She tried several times to talk him into moving, but all he did was block the door and not say a word. Finally, she gave him an ultimatum. "If you don't move right now, I'm going to push by you," she told him, and without waiting for an answer, she ducked under his arm and shoved him to the side, hurrying past, half expecting him to grab her. "He was much bigger than me, and he wasn't listening to me. I didn't really understand what was happening."

She made it downstairs, and he followed her. By then, she was so shaken, all she wanted to do was get away from him. "I said 'come on Matt, I'm taking you home.' Before we left, he started taking everything out of my fridge and putting it in his backpack. I didn't even care. I just wanted him out of my house." She wouldn't allow him to her house again for over a year. "We'd talk on the phone sometimes, but I didn't let him come around anymore."

The final straw for Matt was the day before New Year's Eve. Because of their altercation, Molly had taken out a restraining order. He wasn't allowed to see her, or make any form of contact with her, for the duration of his probation. Even though they'd broken up, he never got over her. "Why won't she talk to me? All I want to do is talk," he said once.

"Matt, if she wanted you to talk to her, she wouldn't have taken out a restraining order. Don't you realize you'll go to jail if you do?" He was still not taking his meds, and no matter what I said, I could tell he wasn't listening.

"She wants to talk to me, she just won't admit it," he said, as surely as if he could read her mind. The annoying exhilaration had returned and was taking over his thoughts.

That day, he went out with Melissa, who again was coming around, and they went to a party. As she remembered, he was very sad about his break up with Molly and wanted to call her. "I told him, 'you can't do it, man. You can't call her or text her at all. Don't do it.'" But true to form, Matt was not going to be told what to do and decided to send her a text message. The message said simply, "I forgive you."

Seeing this message coming from Matt obviously freaked Molly out, and she immediately reported him to the authorities. Because this was a violation of his probation, he was visited by the Bedford police the very next day.

There was heavy knocking on our front door, which I recognized right away as the police. When I answered, there were two of Bedford's finest waiting with stern looks on their faces. "Mr. Green, is Matthew home?" the larger of the two asked. When I acknowledged he was, he said, "We have a warrant for his arrest for probation violation. He disobeyed the restraining order issued against him, and we have to take him in." He then showed me a copy of the warrant.

I knew this day was coming, but I was no less surprised. I couldn't comprehend why Matt would knowingly violate his probation after all our warnings. He is the smartest dummy I know, I thought angrily. I let the officers in and called up to Matt, who was in his room. "Matt, come down please. You have visitors." He came out of his room right away, apparently thinking it was one of his friends. When he saw the officers waiting, he immediately turned around to head back to his room.

"We'd like to do this without any force, Mr. Green," the officer said.

"I'll go up with you and get him to comply, but please understand, he's not in his right mind." The officers had had dealings with Matt before and were very sympathetic.

"We're aware of his condition, sir. Please tell him not to resist."

Less than five minutes later, Matt was cuffed and led to the squad car parked in the driveway. He didn't put up a fuss of any kind, which was surprising. They took him to the Bedford jail to await transfer to the Summit County jail. Apparently, Molly had moved to Akron to go to school there, and the order was issued in that county.

By New Year's Day, 2011, Matt was sitting in the Summit

County Jail, twenty-six miles from home, and in a full blown manic episode. His behavior while there became so bizarre, they had to wrestle with him to get him to court naked, and strapped to a chair, covered only with a blanket. The struggle caused him to be charged with an additional count of aggravated assault on a police officer (one of them broke a finger). He wouldn't talk to anyone, and remained mute for two months. Finally, after repeated tries to get him to speak, his court appointed lawyer filed a motion to have him hospitalized, under court supervision of course, until he was competent enough to assist in his own defense. "Your honor, he won't even talk to me." The attorney sounded frustrated.

As Matt had predicted to his brother, he wouldn't have to spend time in the general population with the other inmates. He was sent to the North Coast Behavioral facility in northern Summit County and would spend the next seven months getting the treatment he so desperately needed, until such time as he was able to converse with his lawyer.

I hate to admit it, but those nine months were the most peaceful Lynda and I had in a long time.

CHAPTER 24

No Mas, Matt

Maybe I need a break, it's true. Maybe I need a break from you. I think you think I know we need one too... or three.

Matt Green, notebook journal 2010

Matt was released from jail in September of 2011 after agreeing to a plea deal with the Summit County prosecutor. He would plead guilty to one felony count of assaulting a police officer with time served, and three years of supervised probation. His lawyer advised him to take the deal because if he went to trial, a jury could find him guilty. He could be sentenced to up to seven years in prison. "You never know what a jury will do," he told us.

Matt, of course, wanted to take it to trial... at first. But after spending the last nine months locked down, he was ready to come home. "I'm just ready to get this over with," he said. Originally, he was supposed to report to a probation officer in Akron, but because he couldn't drive, he was allowed to report to the Bedford probation office since he was still "on paper" there too.

Once again, he told his PO he wasn't going to stop smoking, and again he was told he wouldn't be tested as long as he made his weekly calls to report in. It never ceased to amaze me how Matt could work the system to his advantage. Whenever he got into legal trouble, somehow he'd use his mental illness to work in his favor to get the lightest forms of punishment. "I've never seen anybody with a felony conviction not have to physically report to his PO, and never get tested," Eddie told me incredulously. "Who does that?"

We were all happy to see him come home, especially me. I'd gotten tired of going to the behavioral facility every Sunday, even though I couldn't imagine not going. I had to see his progress from the treatment he needed, and to hear him talking rationally again from the effects of it. I'd bring him pizza and other personal items they'd allow, and we'd play a few games of chess before I'd leave. However, each time we parted, I felt as if I should be taking him home. "My son shouldn't be here," I thought, "but I know it's for his own good." Lynda would go too sometimes. But she couldn't stand to see him in that facility every week. "I'll go, but it won't be every week," she told me. "But when I don't, please tell him I love him and miss him." Again, I was reminded of the vow I'd made to myself years before, of never letting her have to be the one to handle Matt's "issues."

Now that he was home, we had a little celebration with all of his favorite foods, with hugs and kisses all around from his siblings. However, he wasted no time calling up his friends to let them know he was free. In fact, that evening, less than four hours after he was released, one of them came by to pick him up. I was a little jealous that he didn't want to spend at least the whole first day out of jail with us, but I knew deep down, he really wanted to catch up with his friends. "I'll be back early, dad. I just want to kick it with my friends for a while." He got no argument from me. After all, I'd seen some of them coming to visit him at the facility. I appreciated his loyal friends.

As the days went by, it didn't take long for him to start going out with them, not coming home until late at night. This caused Lynda and I to think he was back to his old ways. However, he was taking his meds regularly and keeping his doctor appointments, so I didn't feel we needed to be overly concerned at this point. One thing we were really happy about was his rejuvenated interest in playing his guitar.

He had hooked up with an old friend from his punk years, Chiachi Kornis, who used to play with Criminal Authority, and started recording music. "I went to a recording school in 2009, and when I got out, I had some money which I invested in a project studio. I wanted to record, but I needed practice. The first person I thought of was Matt."

"We'd been in contact on and off, and it was during that time when we were recording that we got pretty close. We became, like best friends. We got back together when he got out of jail." Matt taught Chachi how to play bass lines to his guitar rhythms, and once he got those down pat, Matt would go into his guitar solos. "When Matt played his guitar solos, I'd close my eyes and pretend it was me playing. He was phenomenal!"

At the time, Matt was really getting into his "look." He had grown his hair into an impressive Afro, and he was now sporting a full beard and mustache, which he would never consider shaving off. His attire was usually GQish, and he was constantly perusing issues of the magazine, looking for something different. He wore a pocket watch on a chain with his skinny jeans and sometimes wore a wrist watch along with it. "I want people to know I always know what time it is," he'd say jokingly. His wide leather belt was worn with the buckle to the side because "that's the way the English punks wear them." He'd purchased an army green canvas coat, which he wore all the time, no matter what else he had on.

As Chiachi would tell me later, "Matt had this cool look about him. He had his own style. I remember we were about to record once, and I gave him some expensive headphones to put on. He tried putting them on in different ways so he wouldn't mess up his hair, but they kept falling off. He made me get ear buds, even though the sound quality wasn't as good. He insisted because of his hair."

The two of them spent a lot of time together, not only for the music, but because of their interest in real estate. "We'd talk on the phone for hours sometimes. He was really focused on making deals." They'd grown close enough for Matt to be forthcoming about his illness too. "He'd make it known when he was, or wasn't, taking his meds. He wore all of his flaws on his sleeve. He'd apologize for his moods, which I didn't think was necessary. But that's what was cool about Matt. He didn't care that you knew he was struggling."

It was during the early months of 2012 that I could see his symptoms starting to reappear. There was nothing obvious, but after years of watching him, I could tell when he was on the verge of another episode. His belligerence had returned, and his ideas about imminent success in real estate were becoming more grandiose. He was obnoxious toward Lynda, and argumentative with me. He wouldn't stay focused on anything more than a few minutes and was impatient when he had to wait for one of his friends to pick him up. "What's taking them so long?" he'd say while looking out windows and pacing the floor.

"Matt, it's only been a few minutes since you hung up the phone. They'll be here", Lynda would say.

"I'll sit on the porch and wait," he would reply, and then I'd see him walking down the street, unable to sit anywhere waiting.

Chiachi could see a difference, but unlike us, he thought it was okay. "Sometimes, he'd be overt in his actions. I was like, this guy has too much energy, and it would be hilarious. It was like he couldn't harness it, but we still played. Other times, you could see him go down, and just go through the motions. But he never stopped playing. It seemed no matter what his mood was, he didn't want to quit playing the music."

Matt was constantly on his phone talking to homeowners, trying to buy or sell their houses, using the knowledge he'd gained from his real estate courses. He'd gotten a tax I.D. number for his business, Evergreen Capital Group, LLC, of which he made himself the CEO. "Dad, I'm going to give you two percent interest in the company, so when I make a million, I'll give you $20,000," he said imperiously. I played along.

"Thanks Matt. And what do I have to do to earn it?"

He was excited to see my interest. "All you have to do is answer any emails I get, and take me to check out houses. I won't work you too hard." He was totally serious.

He even tried to recruit his sister Angel to work for him. "He wanted me to follow his lead, like a kind of assistant type thing. But he could be annoying sometimes." She continued, "He'd order me around and be condescending. He told me once, 'if you don't listen to what I say, I'm gonna fire you,' and I wasn't even getting paid!"

He was walking the hallway at night again, keeping Lynda and I awake, worrying about him. "He's going to end up in the hospital again, Rick," she said, and I agreed. Matt knew we couldn't do anything about it because he was an adult. As long as he wasn't a threat to himself, or others, he was not going to get "locked up."

One day, Lynda called me and said she was going to John's house because Matt had said something that made her frightened. "He told me everybody should be killed except him." I could tell by the tremor in her voice she was very afraid.

"He said what?" I just couldn't believe he'd say something like that to her.

"Yes, he actually said that. I'm going to John's house. I'm not staying there alone with Matt." I heard a car horn blow on her end of the phone, so I knew she had already broke camp and was hightailing it to John's.

"Okay, okay, try to relax." I tried to be reassuring. "Where is he now?"

"When I left, he was in his room." I was already thinking of our next move with Matt. Unbeknownst to her, Matt had made that same remark to me a few days before.

I was in the kitchen having a cup of coffee when he came down and sat at the table across from me. I already knew he was in the midst of an episode, but he'd been able to control the manic aspect of it… just barely. He was fidgeting in the chair and couldn't sit still. He would get up, walk around the kitchen a few times, and sit down again. After watching him do that a few times, I finally said, "Matt why don't you either sit down or get up, and stay up. You're making me nervous."

All this time, he hadn't said a word. He sat down, looked at me, and said, "I think everybody should be killed except me." I was shocked by the lack of emotion in his voice when he said it, but I wasn't going to let him see my consternation.

"Does that include your mother and me?"

Without hesitation he said, "Everybody." Still not sure if I should take him seriously, I continued, "Well if 'everybody' is killed except you, it'll be a pretty lonely place, wouldn't it? You would be the only one alive on the planet." I wanted to see how far he would go.

He didn't say anything, just got up and went to his room. I knew he hadn't been sleeping, and when having an episode, he would say the most outlandish things. However, he'd never talked about people being killed before. I was worried, but I knew he had just given me the out I needed to get him treatment. I would have to go to the Cuyahoga County Probate Court to have him involuntarily hospitalized. We'd done it once before, and Lynda felt guilty about having to do it. I thought it would be a hard sell if I brought it up again.

I decided to not say anything about this, but I definitely was going to watch every move Matt made while in the house. I knew I might be taking a chance, especially with Matt's unpredictability, but I felt I was capable of handling him, physically if necessary, if he tried anything.

But now she was telling me he'd said it to her, and she was obviously frightened of him, so I figured this would be the best time to broach the subject. "I'm going to meet you at John's house, and we're going to get Matt probated again. I know you don't like it, but with him talking about killing, we'll be justified in going that route". Surprisingly, she didn't object.

"Fine, let's do it," and then she hung up.

I got to John's house post haste, and Lynda was already there waiting for me. She looked pretty rattled, but when she spoke, the fear I'd heard in her voice on the phone was gone. "I got out of there as quickly as possible. I didn't feel comfortable in the house with him." That's when I told her about him telling me the same thing a few days earlier. She wasn't too happy. "If you had said something then, we could have done this sooner." I didn't argue, I just wanted to get going. We hurried down to the probate court and were called in to see the magistrate after a short wait.

"Mr. and Mrs. Green, please have a seat." The magistrate was a tall, elegant looking woman with piercing blue eyes that looked like they could see right through you. "I understand you wish to have your adult son probated. Please tell me why." We gave her the whole rundown of what Matt had said to both of us at separate times. She didn't interrupt, only listened intently, writing down notes on a legal pad as we spoke. When we were done, she looked at her notes and said,

"Well, his talk of doing harm to others is enough to get the court involved. I'll place a court order to the Bedford police to have him picked up and taken to the nearest psychiatric hospital for an evaluation." She then instructed me to go home to make sure Matt was there. "If he is, keep him there until the police come. Don't worry. We'll get you the help you need."

As we were thanking her, about to leave, she said, "You folks have apparently been going through this with your son for quite a while. My advice to you is, do not let him live with you again. He's an adult, and even with his illness, he should be taking care of himself. Don't enable him any further. I've seen cases like this many times, and the worst thing you can do is allow him back in your house. He either takes better care of himself, or the courts will do it for him. Good luck."

We left her office knowing she was right. We loved Matt so much, our emotions held us captive to his manipulations. No matter what, we'd always be there for him, so he would use that knowledge to have his way. Now both of us had reached our limit. We were ready to let our 25-year-old son feel some tough love. We hoped the realization he couldn't come home as always after getting treatment would be the cold slap in the face he needed to force him to take better care of himself.

We didn't talk much on the way home, each of us feeling a new resolve. This was it. Once he was taken from our house this time, he couldn't come back.

CHAPTER 25

Are You Your Brother's Keeper?

"This is the perfect neighborhood for Matt."

-Eddie Green-

Matt was picked up and taken to Marymount Hospital again, and for once, he didn't resist. The Bedford policemen who came to get him had dealt with him before, so they were able to talk him into compliance using a friendly approach. Plus, I believe Matt knew he needed help and wanted to get better. This was his way of doing that, without admitting it.

I hadn't told him our plans not to let him come home after his release; I didn't want him to have that kind of anxiety while trying to recover. However, I knew he'd only be there a week, so I had to make some arrangements fast.

First, I enlisted the help of his social worker, Christie Washington. She had worked with Matt for about two years

and had earned his confidence and respect. She seemed to have infinite patience when it came to dealing with Matt and wasn't at all intimidated by his intellectual sparing matches with her. "Matt was one of my better clients," she told me later. "He was well spoken, and highly intelligent. I knew of his disability, but we never talked about it. Matt wanted our relationship to be as normal as possible, and I had no problem with that."

We wanted her to look into group homes in the area where Matt could go, and have supervision over his medications. I knew he wouldn't be happy about it, but we were not letting him back with us. Ms. Washington understood and said she'd start compiling a list of potential locations he might like. "They have some really nice ones not far from here. I know how particular Matt can be, so I'll make sure it's not in a bad neighborhood."

Of course, Matt would never agree to any group home, no matter how nice. His idea of purgatory would be living with others who had "character flaws" worse than his. "I'd rather die than go to a group home," he'd told me once when I'd suggested it. Be that as it may, I had to find accommodations for him quickly, and no matter how diligently she tried, Ms. Washington wouldn't be able to come up with a location in a week. "That's not a lot of time, Mr. Green, but I'll do the best I can."

Desperate for an urgent solution, I decided to do something

I never wanted to do… ask my kids for help. I knew his sisters Danielle and Angel were both married and raising their own kids. Even though I knew they wouldn't deny me, I didn't feel comfortable sending Matt to either of them fresh out of the hospital. Likewise, with his brother John. His hands were full with a wife and four kids of his own. Sending Matt to John wasn't an option, period. That left his brother Eddie. He wasn't married and lived alone in a nice two-family house in the Shaker Square district. Of all the kids, Matt was closest to Eddie. Over the years, they'd developed a tight bond and talked to each other frequently. If anyone could get Matt to take better care of himself, it would be Eddie.

I was hesitant, but I called him anyway. The phone rang a long time, and I was about to hang up when he finally answered. "Hello." He sounded winded, like he'd been running.

"Eddie, I need your help," I said, forgoing the small talk.

"What's up dad?"

"Son, I know this will be asking a lot, but I don't have much choice. Matt is in the hospital again, and he'll be getting out in a week. Lynda and I are at our wits end with him and don't want him living with us right now. Will you let him stay with you, until we can get him other accommodations?"

There was a long silence on the other end of the phone. I didn't realize it, but I was holding my breath, waiting for his answer. Finally, he said, "How long will he have to be here?"

"Hopefully not too long. Maybe a month. Just long enough to give his social worker time to locate a group facility he can go to."

After another long pause, he said, "Okay dad, as long as it's not permanent."

I felt like a huge load had been taken off my shoulders. I was finally able to exhale. "Thanks, Eddie. You have no idea how much we appreciate this." I hung up thinking Lynda would be as happy as I, knowing Matt would be staying with his brother. Even though she knew he couldn't stay with us, she didn't want him going to a place that might trigger another episode this soon after getting treatment. She knew how he felt about group homes.

A week later, I picked Matt up from the hospital. "How are you feeling Matt?" I asked. He looked a little thinner, but his demeanor was much better. The treatment he'd received during his stay seemed to have worked.

"I'm okay," he said. "I'm just ready for some of mom's home cooking." I dreaded having to tell him, but I had to.

"Listen Matt, I'm taking you to Eddie's house to stay with him for a while. Your mother and I need a break from you and your unpredictable behavior. I know you're better now, but what about the next time you have an episode? We're getting older. We can't take the strain of your unwillingness to manage your health better. Maybe being with Eddie will change that."

He didn't say anything, which was surprising. However, I could tell by the way he slumped down in the passenger seat and dropped his head that he didn't like it. We rode in silence until I pulled into our driveway. "Go inside and pack enough to last you a couple of days. I'll get the rest of your things later and bring them to Eddie's house."

He got out of the car and slowly walked to the door of our house, then before going in he said, "I'm sorry, dad. I know it's been tough on you and mom, but it's been tougher on me. I just hope you understand."

I almost fell for his guilt trip. It hurt me to have to do this, but I was quite aware of his ability to pull at our heart strings. That sorrowful statement was meant to make me change my mind, but I wasn't about to. Matt was going to Eddie's, and that was that. As I waited for him to pack, Lynda came into the living room and sat next to me. She looked as if she was about to cry, but she wouldn't allow the tears to fall. "Do you think he'll be alright with Eddie? I know they love each other, but that could change once they're living together." She had the same thing on her mind as I did, but I tried to be reassuring. "They'll be fine, and besides, it's only temporary. They'll only have to put up with each other until Ms. Washington comes up with a group home."

"I'm not going to a group home." Matt must have heard me when he was coming down the stairs with his suitcase. "I'll stay with Eddie, but I'll never go to a group home."

"Let's just take it one day at a time, Matt," I said. "Whether you have to go to a group home or not is totally up to you. If you show you can take care of yourself without supervision, there's no reason you can't have your own place. But you have to be responsible enough to keep us from worrying about you."

"I'll show you. I'll get my own place, you'll see." Then he straightened his shoulders and said, "Well, I'm ready. Let's go." With that, he picked up his suitcase and headed out to the car.

As I was leaving, Lynda grabbed my arm and said, "Tell Eddie thanks for me," and gave me a kiss. I could see a single tear come down her cheek, and I gently wiped it away.

"Don't worry baby, this is the best for all of us. It's going to turn out fine."

After stopping to get something to eat, we headed to Eddie's house. The Shaker Square district is a mixture of upscale apartments and restaurants, and the houses are old but well kept. It's at the border of the suburb of Shaker Heights and Cleveland, where old money businesses and urban entrepreneurs coexist.

Eddie's house was a beautiful two-family residence, with a huge front porch, just a few blocks from Shaker Square. He had the two-bedroom first floor, with high ceilings and a brick fireplace in the living room. Being a bachelor pad, the living area was sparse, with a couch, a flat-screen TV, and a long cocktail table. The dining room had a small table with four chairs for eating meals. The bedrooms were small but comfortable. Eddie let us in, gave us both a hug, and sat down on the couch. He'd grown into a well-muscled young man, with powerful looking arms and a broad chest. He'd always been into working out, and it showed.

"Have a seat, dad, while I show Matt his room." They left me in the living room to ponder the situation. I was deeply indebted to Eddie for taking up this new responsibility, but as an ex-Marine, I knew he would be up for the task. Now, the real work was about to begin. Eddie would have to be Matt's caretaker for at least the next month. If Matt was true to form, he'd either get better, or he'd allow himself to have another episode, erroneously thinking that would get him back home. I would give Eddie all the assistance I could by phone, but he would have to see, first hand, Matt's erratic mood swings and how difficult they were to handle.

Eddie came back into the living room alone. "Matt said he was tired and wanted to get some sleep," he said.

"I imagine he does need to sleep, so let him get as much as he wants," I said, and then I got down to the meat of our conversation.

"Eddie, I know you're aware of Matt's illness. You've been around him long enough to know what he's capable of. Right now, you are the one who's going to have to monitor him, and make sure he takes his meds on schedule. Lynda and I didn't have much success getting him to do that. I'm hoping maybe you will be able to get the results we couldn't. He's doing better now, but maintaining his regimen will require you to stay on him. Not like a parent, but as his brother. Whatever that entails, I'm counting on you to find out."

"Well, it's only for a month, so I think I can handle it for that long. But if I need help or advice from you, will you be there?" I could see he was somewhat apprehensive.

"Of course. Anytime you need me, by all means, give me a call." He seemed to relax a little, and took a deep breath.

"Well, I guess it's up to me now, but you know what? I'll just treat this like a lab experiment. I know that sounds crass, but that's the only way I can handle this. Matt's my brother, but he'll try to use his brain to manipulate the situation. I'm gonna have to put him in a kind of boot camp, and he probably won't like it. That's the way it's gonna be."

Eddie, by nature, has an aggressive personality. He has one of the strongest wills I've ever seen. When he puts his mind to something, he usually gets positive results, but he has to be motivated to commit. Having his baby brother under his jurisdiction, although unexpected, was somewhat welcome to him. This gave him something to focus on, and as he said, his "experiment" would be the center of that focus.

Matt was about to meet his match. After a month with Eddie, he might not think a group home was such a bad idea.

CHAPTER 26

Enlightenment

"My friend...care for your psyche...know thyself, for once we know ourselves, we may learn how to care for ourselves"

-Socrates-

PART 1

Six months later, by the fall of 2012, Matt and Eddie had settled into a comfortable coexistence. Although the initial arrangement was only supposed to be for a month, a couple of things happened that changed everything.

First, Matt had another episode two weeks after moving in with Eddie. "Dad, Matt's acting weird, and I don't know what to do. Will you come over?" I'd never heard Eddie sound so unsettled.

"I'm on my way."

I hurried to Eddie's wondering how Matt had gotten sick

again so quickly. I knew his last stay at the hospital was short, and his state of mind was still fragile, but I thought once he got with his brother, he'd do what was necessary to keep himself on an even keel. Eddie had assured me he was taking his meds every day, as prescribed, so how could Matt have relapsed already?

I pulled up to his house and ran to the front door. Eddie was waiting for me with the door open. "Where's Matt?" I asked.

"He's in the dining room, and he won't stop dancing around." He had a worried look on his face. I walked into the house, and I immediately saw Matt. He was moving around the room doing some strange dance. His arms were doing the "wax on, wax off" thing from the Karate Kid, as if he was blocking punches. His upper body is twisting and turning, while his legs and feet moved as fluidly as Michael Jackson doing the moonwalk.

"Matt, what's going on?" I wanted to see how his conversation would be… if I could get him to talk. Sometimes, during episodes, he wouldn't talk at all. Other times, he'd talk total nonsense. Which would it be now?

He looked at me and smiled, never stopping his gyrations, and said, "What's up dad? I'm feeling the groove. Can't you feel it too?" By now, he was moving all around through the dining room and living room, covering his mouth while dancing, and when he removed his hand, his tongue would be sticking out, wagging back and forth.

"No Matt, I don't feel the "groove," but I think we should go see your doctor. Have you been taking your medicine?"

"I'm right as rain, dude," he said, dismissing my question. I turned to Eddie and asked him the same question.

"Has he been taking his meds?" Eddie looked a little uncomfortable and said, "He's been taking his meds on his own. I didn't think he needed me to hand them to him."

That was it! Eddie allowed Matt to be his own monitor. I knew if left to his own devices, Matt would stop taking his meds, and wait for that "annoying exhilaration" to take over. From the looks of it, he hadn't taken his meds since he got there. Now, I had to get him stabilized again, by taking him back to the hospital. I went up to Matt and grabbed him by the arms to stop him from dancing. He seemed a little startled, and I could see a look of apprehension in his eyes.

"Listen, Matt. I'm going to take you back to the hospital so you can get better, but I need you to calm down first. Where's your medicine?" He jerked away from my grasp and danced into his bedroom, with me following close behind. He stopped in front of his dresser and pointed to two full medicine bottles.

"There they are, but I'm not taking them. I don't need to anymore." He then danced out of the room, listening to music only he could hear.

There was no use trying to persuade him to take the medicine now, so I tried another tactic. "Hey Matt, I know where a hospital is with some very pretty nurses. Would you like to check it out?" He stopped dancing and eyed me suspiciously.

"Where is it?"

"Marymount," I said.

He gave me a sneer and said, "I've been there, and those nurses are not pretty." Then he started dancing again. "Maybe not, but I think your friend Alicia may be there," I lied.

Matt had never forgotten his "ice queen." He talked frequently about how they'd pulled off their illicit assignation at St. Vincent Charity a couple of years ago. He said if given the chance, and if they happened to be at the same facility, they'd do it again. At the mention of Alicia, he stopped dancing and said, "Let's go."

All this time, Eddie watched silently as I got Matt to calm down somewhat. Finally, he said, "Hey dad, if you want me to go with you, I will."

PART 2

Matt knew his father was lying, but he didn't care. Something happened during this particular episode that had not happened before.

For about five seconds, at various intervals during the

event (and they were events!), his mind would have absolute clarity, and he could *see* himself acting "weird." For those brief seconds, he saw himself standing on Eddie's couch, gyrating crazily and waving his arms about. This horrified him because he didn't know *why* he was doing it. He'd always imagined himself doing something cool during episodes. Nobody had ever told him otherwise; in fact, a lot of his friends would laugh and play along with his histrionics. However, the knowledge that he could be actually *embarrassing* himself in front of his friends and family, was disconcerting.

Suddenly, as quickly as lucidity came, it was gone. He couldn't remember anything else until the clarity returned some time later. Now, he saw himself prancing around the living room like a ballroom dancer without a partner. However, also in that moment, he saw Eddie sitting on the couch, shaking his head disgustedly, and his dad looking at him with eyes brimming with tears.

Matt was mortified. The two people he respected most were looking at him as if he were an interplanetary alien. In that instant, he could actually see how much his adamancy of doing things his way was affecting his family.

"Oh my God", he thought. "What the fuck am I doing? I've got to stop this." Without warning, he blacked out again… but not totally. He could still see what he was doing, but now it seemed like he was having the most fun he'd ever had… ever! He knew he should stop dancing, but he didn't want to.

"Why aren't they having as much fun as me?" he thought in his altered mental state.

Bam! He was back to seeing clearly. He didn't know how long it had been, but at that moment, he heard his father's Alicia entreaty. Matt knew while he had a few seconds, he'd better hurry up and respond, before he blacked out again. "Let's go," was all he was able to get out before it happened. Back to dancing merrily.

Matt desperately wanted help.

PART 3

Matt got the treatment he needed, spending ten days in the hospital. When he got back to Eddie's, they had developed a tacit agreement. Eddie would administer Matt's meds as prescribed. In return, Matt made sure he took them while his brother watched. "I don't want to have another episode and look like a fool in front of everybody. I never want my friends to see that again," he told Eddie.

"Matt was serious about taking his meds," he recalled. "He used to argue about how he didn't need it, but when he found out he could be embarrassing himself in front of Sam, or Colleen, or any of his Bedford crew, he stopped arguing." Then he said, "Besides, he knew this was his last chance. If he had another episode for noncompliance, he was going to a group home."

A month later, in May of 2012, I became Matt's legal guardian. Neither of us wanted this initially. Matt, of course, didn't want any parental involvement with his personal life. By the same token, I wanted him to be able to fend for himself, and do what was necessary, health wise, to make that happen. We both wanted the other to be free of any worries where his independence was concerned.

However, after several hospital stays, and his inability to keep his illness managed on his own, I felt it was time to step up and help my son in the best way I knew how. With Eddie's influence, I was able to get Matt to go along with the guardianship, with the caveat that I was only responsible for the medical aspect of his life. I would take him to all of his doctor appointments, make sure his medication prescriptions were filled and delivered to Eddie, and once every week, get a status report.

Most importantly, if he did happen to relapse and wouldn't comply, I had the authority to have him involuntarily hospitalized. Before, as long as he "wasn't a threat to himself or others," I couldn't get him to go for treatment, unless he wanted to go.

Of course, all of this was contingent on he and his brother getting along. In spite of their unconditional brotherly love, each of them had reservations about the other.

A few years ago, when Matt and I were sitting by a late evening fire in our backyard fire pit, he told me candidly how he felt about being on his own. "You know something, dad? I don't think I could live by myself. But I don't want a roommate. I wish me and Eddie could live together, but he's way too bossy! I don't like to argue, but he doesn't know how to dial it down to a debate. It would be great if we could have some deep conversations, but I know it won't happen if we live together."

As for Eddie, his skepticism was over Matt's sometimes imperious attitude. Being a former high school wrestler, and an ex-Marine, he was not going to let his little brother lord over him. "Matt is a genius," Eddie once said, "But the fact that he knows it, makes him a selfish asshole sometimes. He's an opportunist who thinks only about himself."

However, after the trauma of the last episode, and the realization that with compromises they could make it work, they found the living arrangements mutually beneficial. Slowly, they started updating their living space. Matt was used to having certain amenities: cable TV, internet access, and a land line telephone. Eddie had been living a Spartan existence, having none of the things Matt had become accustomed to. However, with their combined incomes, within a few weeks, they had not only gotten the cable, internet, and phone, but also had a few more pieces of furniture.

As their sister Angel would put it, "At first, Matt moving

in with Eddie was like Carlton Banks was in the hood visiting. Like he was staying with the help for a minute. But once Matt realized Eddie didn't have the 'basics,' he made it a point to upgrade the house. Matt made Eddie come out of the cave."

As the months went by, the talk of Matt going to a group home was suspended. By the end of 2012, they were comfortably ensconced in their new lifestyle. Even the neighbors were becoming fond of Matt. He'd made friends with the next-door neighbors and was especially close to one of them, Paul Sistrunck, a tall young man, well over six feet, and like Matt, a Capricorn. He was several years younger than Matt, but that didn't stop them from becoming fast friends. "Matt was like a mentor to me," said Paul. "He would always encourage me to follow my dreams, and to prepare for success. He was so passionate about real estate, and knew all about it. One thing about him, he was all about teaching. He loved to show people what he knew."

One day, while I was there visiting (sitting on a new couch, by the way), I asked Matt how he liked living with Eddie so far. He took a moment, but then he said, "He's okay, I guess. He's still bossy, but I'm getting him to actually have decent conversations with me. He even takes my advice sometimes. It's not as bad as I thought it would be."

An added bonus for him was the artsy atmosphere in the Shaker Square District. There were quaint little coffee shops peppered throughout the neighborhood, as well as outdoor festivals held annually during the summer. Cozy restaurants with outside patio dining were prevalent, all within bike riding distance from the house. "I even found some places I can play my guitar, or have a chess game or two," he told me. "I really like this neighborhood!"

All the while, Eddie kept a close eye on his brother. Their brother, John would visit often, as he worked at a barbershop a block away. "Sometimes, Eddie would stay home rather than go out, just to make sure Matt took his meds on time," he said.

Something else developed within Matt that was never acknowledged until his move with Eddie. It was a newfound appreciation of his own African American race. From the time he'd been in Bedford until his arrival at Eddie's, Matt's friends were predominately white. Years of enduring ridicule from black kids because he acted "too white" made him feel they weren't as culturally evolved as he was. He didn't dislike them; he was just disappointed they weren't more open-minded in their thinking. Consequently, he gravitated to those he felt were "on the same page as me."

However, once he'd spent some time at Eddie's house and was able to be around, and know, more black people personally, he began to change his outlook on his ancestry. "I'm associating with people I didn't used to associate with too much. But now, I'm finding out they aren't so bad," he told me. I was pleased to hear him say this, but I still wanted to get a "dig" in.

"Now don't you feel a little guilty for categorizing a whole race of people... your people?"

"I do feel a little bad about that, especially when I talk to somebody like the professor. He's an intellectual like me."

The "professor," whose real name is Michael McCord, is an old-school, street-smart black man with a wealth of knowledge, and like Matt, loved to talk about philosophy. He was also Paul Sistrunck's uncle.

"Almost every day, Matt would come by to talk. He had a curious mind, and was a good listener," said the professor. "Sometimes, we would talk for hours, and neither of us knew we'd been talking that long."

Another advantage to Matt's "associations" was how he was able generate a little extra money by gambling. The professor's brother Ronald, aka "Head," was a dice shooting expert. From years of practice, he knew all the tricks of the trade, and Matt was his very eager student. "Matt loved to gamble, but he wasn't that good. After Head showed him what to do, Matt started taking people's money shooting dice," said Eddie. "I was impressed enough to let him show me. Now, I'm pretty good too."

I was glad to see Matt finally allowing himself to appreciate his heritage, but more than that, Lynda and I were happy to see him managing his health better. Other than when he first got there, he hadn't had another episode in months while with his brother, and we were holding out hope he'd make it through the rest of the year. We all had to remain vigilant, especially Matt. His future depended on it.

CHAPTER 27

Dog Days

"We got a dog!"
-Matt Green-

PART 1

For most of my adult life, I've owned a dog. Not just any dog, but Great Danes. I was always enthralled by their great size and their mild temperament. Great Danes, to me, were the epitome of the kind of dog a family man would want— large enough to be intimidating, but gentle with children. They are very intelligent and easy to train, so when we moved to Bedford, I knew there would be another of these gentle giants roaming the Green household.

I wanted a black Great Dane, the main reason being Lynda didn't want dog hair visible on our new dark carpeting. She figured if any shedding were to happen, black hairs wouldn't be as apparent when visitors came. After attending a dog show and seeing the magnificent black Danes on display with their shiny coats, I knew that was the dog for us. After doing some research, I settled on a breeder who specialized in black Danes.

Lynda, Matt, and I visited the farm where the dogs were being raised, and once in the pen where the puppies were being kept, we were immediately surrounded by five or six Great Dane puppies. Their tails were wagging, and they all seemed to be trying to get one of us to play with them. I stood back to watch the action, and noticed one of the puppies wouldn't leave Lynda's side. Wherever she went, he was close behind. He was the largest of the litter and didn't seem to be as feisty as the others; however, unlike his siblings, he carried himself in an almost regal manner. For a puppy a few weeks old, he seemed wise beyond his years. I knew then this would be the one for us.

Onyx, so named because of his shiny black coat, took to our family right away, and soon became a beloved and trusted addition to our home. Matt spent a lot of time with him, even helped in his training. He enjoyed taking him for walks around the neighborhood and watching the stares from people as he passed by. Matt loved having Onyx, and was proud to be his owner. Over the years, they had become quite a pair. The tall slim rocker, with his black gear and sunglasses, and this huge black dog, standing almost to his waist on all fours. Just about everyone in Bedford knew Matt and Onyx.

The only drawback from owning Great Danes is that their lifespan isn't very long. One would be lucky to get ten years with the dog. We'd had Onyx for about eight years when Matt was incarcerated in the Summit County jail. Our beloved Onyx was getting old; the hair around his snout was just about all gray now. He was becoming incontinent, and had developed hip dysplasia, a common occurrence in large breed dogs. He was having trouble going up and down stairs, and his constant soiling of the carpet made it impossible for us to keep him. With heavy hearts, we decided it was time to let him go. We found a Great Dane rescue farm that was willing to take him, where he would be around other Danes in their golden years.

Matt was upset to find "the loyal hound" wasn't greeting him at the door when he was eventually released nine months later. "You should have tried to keep him, dad. I would have helped," he said.

"We couldn't, Matt. He was getting old and cranky. I didn't want to have him put down. At least his quality of life will be better at the rescue farm." I felt just as bad as he did.

"We have to get another dog, we have to," was all he said. I suspected Matt was vowing to himself he'd have a dog of his own one day. He never mentioned it again.

During the summer of 2013, Matt and Eddie had been roommates for over a year. He'd made friends all over the neighborhood and had even found a young lady to spend time with. Rose Winters was cute in a "girl next door" way, with a sing-song voice that always sounded as if she were asking a question. They happened to be sitting on the porch together when Matt's friend, Paul came by with a puppy.

"Hey Matt, would you mind watching him for me until I come back?" he asked. Matt was a little hesitant because sometimes Paul wouldn't come back right away, and he knew Eddie didn't want a dog in the house. He didn't mind babysitting; he just didn't want to have to explain to his brother why the dog was still there if Paul didn't show up.

"Ok dude," Matt said, "But you have to come back; if you don't, I'm keeping him." Matt was bluffing, but only half-heartedly. He really did want to keep the dog, but Eddie had made it abundantly clear there were to be no pets in the house. But the little pit bull terrier was so cute and full of energy that Matt loved him at first sight. Since Paul had moved next door with his uncles, they wouldn't allow him to keep his puppy there either. So he would bring him over and let Matt play with him, hoping he and Eddie would take him in. Matt decided if Paul didn't come back, he would have to convince Eddie to keep him.

As Rose would tell me later, "Paul asked me and Matt to watch the puppy. Matt said okay, but Paul didn't come back for him. We were stuck with the dog. Matt asked me to take him home with me, but I already had three dogs, so I couldn't keep him. That's when Matt decided he'd keep him." Now, he had to figure out a way to convince Eddie to let the dog stay. He'd lived through his brother's tirades before. One more couldn't be that bad, could it?

It was getting dark, and Matt knew eventually he'd have to come up with a plan. Eddie came out of the house and saw them on the porch with the puppy. "I'm about to leave Matt, but don't bring that dog in the house, you hear?"

"Yeah, I hear you," he said, and watched Eddie hop into a car with one of his friends and pull off.

"What are you gonna do, Matt?" Rose asked him. "I don't know yet, but I'll figure out something."

After Rose went home, Matt began to think of his options. He didn't have many, but the one that made the most sense was to somehow hide the dog until he figured out a way to bring it to Eddie. Once it was completely dark, Matt took the puppy into the house, hidden under his coat. By this time, Eddie had come home, but didn't notice the small bulge protruding from Matt's coat. "I'm tired, Ed. I'm going to bed." And with that, Matt hurried to his room and closed the door.

He hopped in the bed with the puppy and covered up, pulling the blankets over both their heads. The puppy snuggled up to him and went to sleep while Matt stared at the ceiling, worried about what the morning would bring. He finally drifted into a troubled sleep. The last thing he thought of was how angry Eddie would be when he found out. But he ultimately didn't care. He'd already made up his mind he was keeping this dog.

PART 2

Since they'd lived together, Eddie had a habit of going into his brother's room every morning so he could, "fuck with Matt." He burst through the bedroom door, hoping to startle Matt, but he was the one who ended up startled. First, Matt's head popped out from under the covers. Then, as if on cue, the puppy peaked his head out and started to lick Matt's face.

Eddie was caught off guard. The last thing he expected to see was this dog in the house. "Matt, I thought I told you not to bring him in here. Are you serious?" Oh shit, the jig was up! Matt hadn't planned on dealing with Eddie so soon. All he could think of was to play to his compassion.

"Come on, Ed. Paul couldn't keep him, and he didn't have anywhere else to go. I wasn't going to put him out on the streets. Look at him, Eddie. He's so cute. We gotta keep him."

Eddie grabbed the puppy by the scruff of his neck, lifting him to eye level. "I don't want this mutt shittin' all over the house."

Matt was insistent. "Come on, Ed. I'll take care of him. You won't have to do anything, because he'll be my dog."

Eddie stared at the little ball of fur for a long time, then said, "We'll keep him for now, but I'm gonna see if I can sell him. I don't want no dogs around here." Matt was ecstatic.

"We got a dog, we got a dog!"

However, things apparently didn't go that smoothly. According to Paul, there was a lot of commotion going on next door. "The next morning, I could hear Eddie yelling at Matt about the dog. Later that morning, Matt came out smiling and said, 'Eddie punched me for that, man.'" Even Rose commented on Eddie's verbal thrashing. "It was so funny because Matt did a great imitation of Eddie using all these cuss words at him and the dog. It was hilarious!"

Whatever abuse he had to take from Eddie, verbal or otherwise, must have been well worth it. He'd accomplished his mission. He'd withstood the wrath of his brother, and had somehow convinced him to keep the dog. After a few months, Eddie wasn't talking about selling him anymore. He'd actually taken over the training of the puppy, who Matt had named Cain, and regularly took him on long walks. Once he was house broken, Eddie started to enjoy having Cain around.

In October of that year, after eighteen months of living with Eddie, Matt wanted to come home. He hadn't had an episode the whole time, and he was working hard to maintain his mental health. He'd even started an exercise program because he'd heard it could stave off depression. Lynda and

I saw the progress he'd made, and were impressed with his newfound maturity. We decided to let him move back in with us.

However, Matt wanted to bring Cain too. We weren't eager to have another dog in the house, but since Matt assured us he would be the one to take care of him, I said "okay." But I gave him an ultimatum. "I've seen Eddie with Cain, and I'm not sure he'll want him to leave. Tell him he has 48 hours to decide if he's going to keep him or let him come with you. If he doesn't make a decision in two days, I'll make it for him. The dog stays where he is. You have two days."

Needless to say, Cain stayed with Eddie, and is with him to this day. The puppy he didn't want is now his constant companion. The irony wasn't wasted on Matt. "Who would have thought Eddie would be that attached to Cain, after all the shit I had to go through to keep him. Now he's Eddie's dog, and I'm back to not having one again."

In hindsight, I'm glad it turned out that way.

CHAPTER 28

Now I Lay Me Down to Sleep

"Sometimes my dreams are so good, I don't want to wake up."
-Matt Green-

On October 14th, 2013, I was helping Matt move his things back into his room. After living with Eddie, he'd become a different person from the one we'd banished from our home eighteen months ago. His maturity was immediately obvious because, for one, he didn't have anything bad to say about his time away, nor the reason why it had to happen in the first place. We both knew, without having to say it, this was the last straw. The dawning of this realization was what I attributed to his new attitude.

"Hey dad, you have no idea how happy I am to see this bedroom!" he said as he loaded his books back on the shelves that had remained empty during his absence. "The next time I leave this room, it's gonna be on my terms."

I watched as he methodically looked at the spine of each of his many books and carefully placed them, much like a seasoned librarian, according to their theme. "You can't put Shopenhauer next to Ayn Rand, and you can't put either of them next to Hunter S. Thompson," he said.

Lynda and I were so happy to see our son healthy and focused. He was still staying on track with his meds and doctor appointments, going so far as to have his social worker drive him when he needed to get a ride. "I'm doing much better, and I know it's because of the 'beans.' But you'll have to take Eddie's place, and give them to me dad. I know I'll stop if you leave it up to me." This new maturity was a pleasant surprise!

"No problem, Matt. I'll be happy to make sure you don't fall of the wagon," I said. He smiled, gave me a hug, and handed me a small bag with his various medications. "Thanks, dad. I know you won't let me down." He then continued to arrange his belongings in their pre-designated places in his room.

I left him thinking this was too good to be true. I really wanted to believe Matt had finally gotten it, and would stay on the straight and narrow. However, we'd had our hearts broken too many times in the past to be more than cautiously optimistic. The one thing that gave me a little solace was knowing I was now his legal guardian. If things went south again, that gave me the authority to take the necessary measures to help him. More importantly, I wouldn't need his permission to do it. I sincerely hoped I wouldn't have to ever use that option anytime soon.

He hadn't had an episode in over a year, and Eddie assured me it was because he made sure Matt took his meds on schedule. "You have to make sure he takes 'em every day, dad," he'd told me. I fully intended to honor that commitment as well as he did.

The first few days back home went well. Matt helped around the house with the chores, something he refused to do before. He also spent a lot of time with Lynda while she cooked up meals in the kitchen. He even came up with a recipe for pasta salad that they worked on together. The result was absolutely delicious, and became a permanent staple in the Green family cookbook.

He still went out with his Bedford gang; someone would come by to pick him up within minutes of his calling them. I think they were happier than we were to see their friend back home and healthy. However, I did notice a difference there as well. Even though he would go out with them, he always made sure they had him home in time for his night meds. "He used to say 'my dad will kill me if I don't get home in time to take my meds,'" said his friend, Colleen Allison. "We were happy to do it because we knew he needed them to stay healthy. He was in a good place, and he wanted to stay there."

I knew sleep was essential to maintaining his mental health, but now he understood the importance of it too. "I need my sleep, dad. That's why I asked the doctor for something to help. She prescribed Ambien. That's the only thing that seems to work." I was somewhat leery of Ambien. I knew it could have some troubling side effects, but if it helped him sleep, I was all for it. That is, until I saw him sleepwalking.

About a month after he'd come home, I was in the living room watching a late-night movie. It was about 2 a.m. when I heard someone walking around upstairs. I thought it might be Lynda getting up to use the bathroom, so I didn't pay it much attention. A few minutes later, I saw a barefoot, shirtless Matt, coming slowly down the stairs in only his pajama bottoms.

"Hey Matt, is anything wrong? Are you having trouble getting to sleep?" I asked. He didn't say anything, just walked right past me, and headed toward the kitchen. As he went by, I could see his eyes were almost completely closed, opened only a slit, and focused on nothing. I immediately thought of the Ambien, and knew he was sleepwalking.

I didn't want to startle him by giving him a sudden shake; I didn't know what kind of reaction that would cause. So I decided to follow him to make sure he didn't hurt himself, but secretly, I wanted to see what he did while in this state.

I sat down in one of the kitchen chairs and watched as he went into the refrigerator. He pulled out a carton of milk, then reached on top of the fridge where we kept all our breakfast cereals, grabbing his favorite, Apple Crunch Cinnamon Cheerios. He shambled over to the cabinet and got a bowl, carrying all three items to the table. He still didn't say anything to me, even though I was sitting right in front of him. In the dim light from the refrigerator (he'd left the door open), I could see his eyes were still semi-closed, but he never bumped into anything while moving around the kitchen.

I sat in amazement as he got a spoon from the utensil drawer, and sat down in the chair across from me. As if on automatic pilot, he poured the cereal into the bowl, poured milk over the cereal, and started eating. Even though he wasn't looking at what he was doing, he didn't overfill the bowl, or spill a drop of milk. "How did he do that?" I thought. He hadn't opened his eyes or moved his head at all during the whole process.

He finished his bowl of cereal, and without a word, poured up another. Once again he didn't make a mess. It was as if some invisible puppeteer was pulling his strings, entertaining me with his deft maneuverings. I continued watching as he finished his second bowl, returned the milk to the fridge, and placed the cereal back on top, finally closing the refrigerator door, (I had intentionally left it open). He turned around and headed back the way he came, with me following close behind. Moving with that slow shuffle, he climbed the stairs, and made it back to his room. I watched him get into bed, and pull the covers up. Within minutes, I could hear him snoring softly.

Damn, that Ambien is some powerful shit! Even though Matt had gone on this nocturnal jaunt and made it safely back to bed, I was still worried by the thought of it happening again. I was lucky enough to be up when it happened, but what about the next time, when I'd be asleep too? Then a terrible thought came into my head. What if he walks outside in the middle of the night? All sorts of horrifying scenarios popped into my mind. I was going to have to talk to his doctor about this as soon as possible.

I sat on the couch, still thinking, the late-night movie completely forgotten. I couldn't relax knowing my son was sleepwalking. I had no idea if it would happen again, but I was going to do what I could to keep him safe. I decided right then I'd sleep on the couch for a while to make sure I'd hear him coming. Being a light sleeper, I knew he couldn't get by me undetected. For the next couple of weeks, if it meant I had to lose a little sleep so he could get his, so be it. I was not going to let Matt have another relapse. He was doing too well with his recovery for me to allow that to happen. Maybe next time I'd have a bowl of cereal with him.

The next day, I headed into the kitchen for my morning coffee. Sitting in the same chair he'd sat in last night was Matt, looking at me suspiciously, holding his box of cereal. "Hey dad, did you eat my cereal? This box is almost empty, and I know I had more than this in here," he said, shaking the box.

I looked closer at him to see if he was joking, but I knew he wasn't. He really had no idea what had happened last night. I didn't say anything right away; I needed my coffee. Unlike him, I didn't get any sleep, walking, or otherwise. He looked at me impatiently, waiting for me to say something. After a couple of sips of the strong java, I finally asked, "How'd you sleep last night, Matt?"

He gave me a curious look and said, "I slept like a rock all night. Now did you eat my cereal, yes or no?"

"Nope, I didn't eat your cereal, but I know who did."

He cracked a smile then and said, "I knew it! Mom ate it. She likes this cereal too." He seemed to be satisfied with his theory, and nodded his head. "I knew it was her." I couldn't hold it back any longer.

"No Matt, it wasn't your mother. It was you."

He stopped smiling, gave me the Gary Coleman, "whatchu-talking-about-Willis" look and said, "What do you mean it was me?" I didn't know how to really explain what had occurred, so I just decided to tell him what I observed. After he heard all the details of his gastric expedition, he looked down dejectedly and said, "I knew it. I knew I'd have some side effects from Ambien, but that's the only thing that helps me sleep."

I could hear the desperation in his voice, so I said, "It's okay, son. Now that I know what to expect, I've decided to sleep on the couch for a while to make sure you won't hurt yourself. Although I have to admit, from what I saw last night, you handled yourself pretty well moving around the house. I didn't have to help you once during that whole time."

He lightened up at that and said, "Really?"

I patted him on the back and said, "Hell yeah! You moved around this kitchen like you were wide awake. You didn't so much as stub your toe."

Things got back to normal after that. I'd slept on the couch for two weeks, and he hadn't done any more sleepwalking of any kind. After a while, I thought it was just an anomaly and wouldn't happen again. I prayed I was right. It was the end of the year, and we were all looking forward to the coming holidays.

Matt, especially, was excited to be home and have some good holiday home cooking. From Thanksgiving, to Christmas, to New Year's Eve, he knew Lynda would make some of the most sumptuous meals he'd ever seen, and couldn't wait to taste. "I'm gonna eat until I pass out," he said. "I love mom's holiday food!"

True to his word, Matt made sure to gorge himself to the point of misery, at all of the aforementioned holidays. He was happier than I'd seen him in years, and he seemed to really enjoy being around his family and friends. I guess he realized how much he missed Bedford, and decided never to take his neighborhood for granted again.

When the ball dropped on New Year's Day of 2014, we were all having champagne and making half-hearted resolutions. When it came time for his, Matt said proudly, "I'm going to be twenty-seven in a few days, and I'm gonna be a millionaire by the time I'm thirty. You just watch." Lynda and I raised our glasses and I said, "To Matt. May all his wishes come true. No one deserves it more." We drank up, and laughed into the night.

Matt turned twenty-seven on January 6, 2014. He had seven more weeks to live.

CHAPTER 29

The Culmination

"Life is a journey that must be traveled, no matter how bad the roads or accommodations."

-Oliver Goldsmith-

Well, we already know how this story ends. I started this journey trying to bring a little understanding of who Matt Green was to his family and friends. However, I believe they actually knew him better than I, so in a way, this story was more for me.

I loved my son more than the air I breathe, but because of that love, I didn't allow myself to see him without my "bipolar-colored glasses." His illness blinded me to the beautiful person he really was. I now know he tried desperately to get me to see his other attributes, and unlike me, to not dwell on his disabilities. So in that respect, I have finally taken off those glasses, and have learned what a truly special son I had.

I know Matt better than I ever did when he was alive, and for that, I will have eternal regrets. However, his presence in our lives has made Lynda and I much closer, and my compassion has been amplified tenfold.

Matt's determination, and courage, to live his life under his own terms and not to listen to the naysayers who were constantly nagging at him made him the "gold standard" for anyone professing to be an individual. As he wrote in his journal in 2012, "The real and genuine individual can always stand alone, and walk freely, without the aid of a tag of any sort. They define the labels others affix, by simply living their lives, and having a lifestyle worthy of that title."

My son was a brilliant and talented man whose self-awareness made him a force to be reckoned with. He knew the importance of acquiring knowledge, even if it wasn't from a college or university. He kept an open mind and never passed judgment on anyone.

Most importantly, he refused to sacrifice his individualism to "fit in." He was truly, as his best friend Sam Sizemore once said, "unapologetically himself." Having said that, I'll relate a poem that I think epitomizes Matt's life, and his philosophy of it. It was written by William Earnest Henley, and it's called "Invictus:"

Out of the night that covers me, black as the pit from pole to pole,
I thank whatever gods may be, for my unconquerable soul.
In the fell clutch of circumstance, I have not winced nor cried aloud,
Under the bludgeonings of chance, my head is bloody, but unbowed.
Beyond this place of wrath and tears, looms but the Horror of the shade,
And yet the menace of the years, finds, and shall find me, unafraid.
It matters not how straight the gate, how charged with punishments the scroll,
I am the master of my fate, I am the captain of my soul.

Thank you, Matthew Thomas Green. I'm so happy, and proud, to have called you my son.

POSTSCRIPT

Since starting this book, a few things of note should be mentioned.

When Matt passed we allowed his corneas to be donated to two people that needed them to improve their vision. The irony of that wouldn't be lost on Matt, and I think he would have approved.

My son John had a fifth child named Rylan Matthew Taylor. It was his way of keeping his brother's memory alive.

Cain the pit bull terrier that Matt "got hit for" has had a family of his own. He sired several puppies in three years and two of them live right next door to Eddie and Cain. Again, I think Matt would enjoy the irony.

Finally, and this was a REAL surprise, I recently discovered I have another son, with three kids of his own! We've started to develop a pretty good relationship, and our family is doing their best to make he, and my new grandkids, welcome. I'm considering this a blessing.

I guess God's sense of humor isn't always cruel.

November 16, 2017

Acknowledgements:

I'd like to thank all the people that helped in the writing of this book.

To those I interviewed, and who allowed me to use their quotes, you have my eternal gratitude. Without your input this would not have been possible.

Sam Sizemore and Colleen Allison, whose insight and anecdotes were integral to completing this endeavor. Thank you both for always being there for Matt.

Thanks to Jesse Carter for his wealth of information about the Gypsy Gipsons and their music, and his unwavering support of this book.

To Joe Revay, Jim Carol, Melissa, and Elizabeth Deal, Greg Slawinski, Malcolm Regan, and Kevin Warner, Matt's loyal inner circle. Your early recollections of Matt and his antics were not only humorous, but very enlightening. Listening to your stories was the fuel that started the engine for me to write this book.

Finally, to my wife Lynda, and my kids, Danielle, Angel, John, and Eddie. Thank you for all your love, patience, and understanding during a most difficult time for all of us. But mostly for not taking "Rick the Prick" too seriously!